Accl

Freedom
from Obesity

*A*s an environmental educator, all too often
I work with kids who don't get to spend enough time
outdoors. Their addiction to digital devices and the
Internet is spawning a new generation of obese youth.
Karen's unique insights can help all children and young
adults find their master key to be free from obesity.

— John C. Robinson, author, *Birding for Everyone*,
www.onmymountain.com

*E*very good teacher was first a good student. Karen
and her husband Dr. Ben Locklear excelled in my mentoring
program, Loral's Big Table (LBT) and are now part of the
LBT Alumni Community. Karen is a passionate teacher
who walks her talk. If you want to drop the weight for
good, read this book immediately. It will change your life.

— Loral Langemeier, Founder/CEO of Live Out Loud, Inc.
and bestselling author.

This is the most powerful, persuasive, and practical book on becoming thin and healthy you will ever read. Page after page, Karen will surprise you with wisdom and refreshing perspectives from her personal journey. Finally ... a practical approach that you can easily apply to your life. Hurry to engage your unique combination and unlock an irreversible change in your health and weight.

— Kim Williams, Certified Stress and Weight Management Health Coach, CEO Vision In Motion Success Coaching. Proudly serving Karen's clients since 2010.

In a world abundant in 'How to,' calorie counters, count your carbs, measuring scales, and numerous other strategies, I find Karen Locklear's philosophy of 'freedom' from obesity refreshing. While other systems for weight reduction might have their place in our society, we need to contemplate the basic philosophy of freedom from obesity and the basic principles of health which this fine work offers—a must read for our culture!

— Marlene Stahl, High School language teacher, Richmond, California

Freedom
from Obesity

*Unlock Your Combination
To a Healthy Weight*

KAREN WARREN LOCKLEAR

LiveOutLoud Publishing

Freedom From Obesity
Unlock Your Combination to a Healthy Weight
Copyright © 2012 by Karen Warren Locklear

http://tlclean.com/

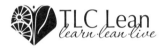

For information, or to order additional copies of this book, please contact:

Live Out Loud Publishing
Phone: 707 688-2848 / Fax: 707 402-6319
Email: info@earnprofitsfromyourpassion.com
Cover and book design by Cypress House

Publisher's Cataloging-in-Publication Data

Locklear, Karen Warren.
    Freedom from obesity : unlock your combination to a healthy weight / Karen Warren Locklear. -- Marysville, Ohio : Live Out Loud Pub.,
c2011.
     p. ; cm.
    ISBN: 978-0-9679338-5-6
    1. Weight loss. 2. Obesity--Psychological aspects. 3. Food habits. 4. Health. 5. Physical fitness. 6. Self-realization. I. Title.
    RM222.2 .L63   2012 2011938526
    613.2/5--dc23 1203

Dedication

This work of my heart is dedicated to the memory of my wonderful grandmothers, Dorfie Short Warren and Lettie Allen Perry. My grandmothers taught me many great lessons in life. They showed me how to live and love abundantly within the confines of an obese body and its associated health problems. Without them I would not have been able to tell my freedom story.

Contents

Acknowledgments

I am truly at a loss for words as I consider the many people who deserve recognition for helping me create this book. There is no way I can properly identify everyone who helped this dream come true. However, I owe much to the legacy I inherited from my parents, CA and Nancy Warren. Words cannot express the amazing transformation that has occurred because of the love and support of my family, and especially my husband Ben. I have truly been blessed with a great family that extends far and wide. I express my appreciation to Loral Langemeier for allowing me to see the greater picture and connecting me with other amazing people. I am thankful to John C. Robinson and the Live Out Loud Publishing team for their constant support in making this become a reality. To those of you who believed in me and supported my vision and dreams, I thank you. Above all, I am thankful to God for His many blessings.

A Note From the Author

I wrote this book for you as if we were having a personal conversation. I want you to know that I wrote from my heart. There are countless self-help books to help those struggling with their weight. I've read a lot of them. They make numerous promises. Experts, authors who hold multiple degrees and are very knowledgeable about their subject matter, wrote many of these books. I want to meet you where you are. If you need to know all the statistics and see the double-blind studies, this book will not meet your needs.

All the stories you are about to read are true. The people in them are letting me share their stories in the hope that you too will soon have a freedom story to share. I love all the people whom I have written about, because I have learned and continue to learn many lessons from them. Their stories are unique to each of them, but have in common that they are what we see happen when people make the changes discussed in this book.

Each of us has a mission in life. I believe mine is to help others unlock their combination to a healthy weight. I am now thankful for having struggled with my weight and health. Every day I am appreciative of my abundant health at a healthy weight. If there had never been any struggles, this book would not have come about. I believe that I am to share my heart with others so I can help them uncover their own hearts. We can do this by shedding pounds and inches.

You won't need to take notes or try to absorb the contents of this book — just sit back and enjoy reading. I am confident you will get what you need from it. My love to you as you find your combination to unlocking your healthy weight. Freedom from obesity is available to you. Look forward to celebrating your freedom.

Freedom
From Obesity

Chapter 1

Freedom Is...

If we were to ask a hundred people to describe what freedom is, we would hear a hundred different answers. The exciting thing is that they would all be right! This understanding is exactly why I love to work with people and help them along their path. It is exciting to see how people can take something and make it uniquely their own.

We often see people who own exactly the same house, with the floor plan and every structural detail alike right down to the doorknobs. Once the families take the first steps into their new houses, a transformation occurs: the houses become homes. No longer are they identical. They become unique, reflecting the character of each individual family. Though identical in foundation and structure, the houses are very different.

We can use this example about anything. No two snowflakes are alike, yet they are definitely snowflakes. I have yet to see a ladybug whose markings are identical to another's.

Do we all agree that we are all very much alike yet uniquely different at the same time? This is a very big concept that must be understood as you read this book. The human design is the same, but to have abundance in our life, we must embrace it as our own. We can honor the design and care for it with all the love we have to give, but at the same time, we must live our lives and show our love through our individuality.

What has this to do with freeing ourselves from obesity? Everything. First we need to discover for ourselves what it is to be truly free. Freedom is as different and unique as the individual. Freedom is a new concept to most people when they are considering their weight issues. Often, strict diets, difficult workouts, and calorie restriction saturates the minds of those who struggle with their weight.

The problem for most overweight and obese people is that they have grown accustomed to being overweight or obese. They have been in bondage so long that they do what they must to accommodate their problem instead of seeing freedom as an option. I am here to tell you that freedom *is* an option. Freedom from obesity can be yours. I have found it, and am excited to help others find their combination to a healthy weight as well.

I believe with all my heart that most people who struggle with their weight are trapped in a belief system that limits their vision of what is truly possible. The purpose of this book is to enlighten you to the fact that freedom is a possibility. You can be free from carrying extra weight and the health and life limitations associated with your weight issues.

While you read this book, keep in mind that this is the story of my freedom experience. Your own freedom experience may be similar, yet it will be uniquely yours. Also keep in mind that if you don't truly believe that freedom is achievable, you will remain bound in your current situation.

Yes, you will make do. Yes, you will adapt, just as you would acclimate to a climate change. Yes, you will be in helpful company, because seeing freedom and reaching for it does take effort. Yes, you will enjoy victories in the bondage.

You can be content in an obese, unhealthy body. I was. I acclimated very well. I had a support team that was happy exactly where they were. We shared the latest and greatest diets, programs, and "miracle cures." What we were missing was a way out. We were missing a view of the possibilities that were available to us. We were missing a belief that we could live free from our unhealthy lifestyle. We were missing our own combination to unlock a healthy weight.

An old pair of shoes may be comfortable, but they aren't the best available. We all have a favorite item that we can't seem to let go of. My husband has a robe that is over twenty years old. It has holes. It is worn thin. It's just ugly. Family members have bought him nice new robes, but which robe does he choose to wear? That old, worn-out, ugly robe is always his pick. He is so bound to his habits that he can't see the benefit of change. Yes, change can be hard, even when it's for the better.

We all experience this struggle with holding on to what is comfy and familiar. This is a factor when it comes to our weight and health issues as well. We are more comfortable with the familiar state we are in. Change, even though it would be in our best interest, is just too hard. When I have the privilege of working with others, this is a central part of the challenge. We have hopes of being lean and healthy, and we make attempts to be free, but our successes are brief.

I understand this concept too well. So often, I tried ways to free myself from bondage. From time to time I experienced a smaller body size or a reduction in weight, but my freedom was short-lived; I always returned to the comfortably familiar prison of my unhealthy body.

The purpose of this first chapter is to entice you. I want you to know what freedom is for me. I want to touch you where other things have not — your heart. I will have accomplished my first goal if you can see what freedom from obesity truly is. These are my highlights.

Freedom is:

* Never buying or struggling with Queen-Sized Control-Top Pantyhose again.
* Never buying clothes with "Big Mama" or "Big Women" on the tag.
* Tying my shoes in one try, without having to come up for air to get the job done.
* Not needing to lie on the bed and kick till my jeans are on and zipped.
* Eating anything I want and knowing it is good for me.
* Craving foods that fuel my healthy, vibrant body.
* No longer craving foods that aren't best for me.
* Chasing *and catching* a sheet of paper that the wind has carried away.
* Running and playing with my grandchildren, without limitations.
* Choosing clothes based on color, fabric, and design instead of size.
* Knowing that my shapely body will fit beautifully into designer clothing.

- Being able to breathe freely while I try on clothes in front of a full-view mirror.
- Knowing people see the "real me".
- Enjoying a meal with friends and family, without concern about what I can and can't eat.
- Attracting more friends to share an abundant life with.
- Enjoying exercise and reshaping my body with weights. Yes, I said *enjoying exercise!*
- Loving to care for and clothe my remodeled body.
- Dressing up for special occasions.
- Enjoying being in public and around new places and people.
- Wearing the same-size clothing and not fluctuating depending on the day or time of the month.
- Liking the first thing I put on in the morning.
- Tucking in and belting, and wearing necklaces as belts.
- Borrowing clothes from a petite teenager.
- Being mistaken for a much younger woman.
- Being asked about body care and health issues.
- Shopping, and finding that everything fits properly and looks good.
- Having much more energy to serve others.
- No longer feeling limited by aches and pains and allergies.
- Having a body that supports health instead of illness.
- Knowing what to eat to support my healthy body.
- Developing healthy habits for a very rewarding life.
- Knowing these changes can last a lifetime.

◆ Enjoying an abundance of food choices.

◆ Not suffering from the problems common to the obese: high blood pressure, high cholesterol, diabetes, fibromyalgia, chronic fatigue, menstrual problems, and breast tenderness.

◆ Enjoying balanced moods and much more pleasure and happiness.

◆ Enjoying a daily routine that supports my healthy weight.

◆ Happy to be in photos instead of hiding behind the camera as the family photographer.

◆ Enjoying enhanced intimacy with my husband. (Of interest to men: The answer is *yes* — there's no need for pharmaceutical enhancement. My husband is also free from obesity and enjoying a healthy life.)

◆ Abundant joy in knowing that I'm free for life.

The greatest freedom is to just be me — the person God designed me to be. I'm free to make my life the best it can be because I am no longer limited by a body that is not mine. Yes, it was a body I created by the decisions I made. That's where the freedom comes in: I now know better and know I can do better.

Has my long list of freedoms captured your attention? I want you to see freedom from your weight struggles as a real possibility. I hope you will let me help you in finding freedom. I would be overjoyed if you received the help you're looking for. The greatest blessing will be when many find their personal combination to a healthy weight and become free from obesity.

Did you find anything on my freedom list desirable? Can you express being free? I have been in both places: The majority of my life was spent in bondage, my whole adult life limited by health issues. I did good things, and I achieved much, yet I was still limited because of my obesity. I won't say that I was miserable. I was very content. After all, I was in good company. My husband was obese, and so were my parents. My children were affected because of the choices I made and the habits I formed. We were content, not because we had no other choice but because we didn't *know* we had a better choice.

Most people aren't aware that they can be free. They don't realize that they can get off the roller coaster of dieting. They don't know of anyplace where a new weight-loss plan, program, or product isn't offered every day. Having permanent freedom is never offered as an option. Our attitude is: *This is the way it is, so live with it.* Or, we might think, *it could be worse, so be content where you are.*

Well, I wasn't content. I dreamed of being free. I remembered having been free as a young girl. It was a wonderful place, and I desired to go back there. Limitations were few. Unlimited possibility was within my grasp. My weight wasn't even a thought, let alone an issue.

I knew deep down in my soul that freedom from obesity was possible because I had experienced it long ago. I had friends and family who did not struggle with weight issues. What was I missing? I had tried it all. There had to be an answer.

The answer is not just one thing. It's like the house, the snowflake, and the ladybug. The answer is as uniquely different as the individual. It's not just some magic pill or product. No one can sell the complete answer in any one program. You need a plan designed specifically for you — a combination of right answers, your individual answers, your combination to a healthy weight is available to you.

This might sound difficult or even impossible. It might seem like a lot of work. You might feel it's not worth the trouble. These could be your feelings if you've been in bondage for a long time and are comfortable where you are. I understand those feelings. At one time I felt all of them, but I no longer do.

I'll never go back to the confinement of a body that is not mine. I will not be limited anymore. I know I could go back, but I will not go back. I will not live that way any longer. I love being free! I love helping others gain their freedom. It is extremely rewarding to be surrounded by those who are free. My husband, my parents, and many of my friends are enjoying the new paradigm, living a healthy life at a healthy weight.

It is not a pipe dream. You can be free. It's all up to you. Are you ready to make your list of "freedom is"? It is not easy, but it's worth it. *You* are worth it! You deserve to be free from obesity.

If you're ready, I'm happy to be your guide. This isn't a "how-to" plan; it's more of an investigation process, and it's more fun than hard. I know you're ready.

First, let's walk down my path. Then we'll learn the basics, and then you will find your combination. Don't forget: I know some good shortcuts. There will be things that are familiar. There will be things you did once but have forgotten. You will be reminded of what has worked and what hasn't. Above all, you'll be amazed at how you transform your life when you find freedom from obesity.

Chapter 2

Free from Obesity

In the United States today, authorities report an over-weight/obesity rate of 70%. Some researchers show data indicating this statistic may be closer to 80%! I think we would all agree we have a problem. Unhealthy weight is contributing to a cascade of health problems. In the US alone, $160 billion are spent on these problems each year. My intent is not to discuss the problems or give a list of resources that hash and rehash the trouble with being overweight. My goal is to give you hope. If you are reading this, and you fit the statistics for unhealthy weight, you already know the consequences. You deal with them every day in every way. I have yet to meet a person in this situation who didn't want to find a way to be free from the bondage of obesity. I have met people who had given up trying for freedom or a way to break the bondage of obesity, which I understand to my core. I understand because I struggled in this prison for forty years.

I want you to know that there is an answer. It is not in a pill, product, exercise, food, or program. The answer is within you. You hold the combination to the lock. I admit it might sound crazy, but think about it. If what we were doing was working, we would all be at a healthy weight and you would not be reading this book. You are a very special and unique individual, as unique as your fingerprint. The key is in the combination that is correct for you. If you're like me, you've tried everything. You may be on the right track, but haven't yet found the correct combination. When someone tells you they have The Key, be cautious. Remember: there is no magic solution that will work for everyone. Is there a combination that's right for you? Is it possible that one day you can declare yourself free from obesity? I believe the answer is yes to both questions.

I grew up in a rural farm community and attended a very small school. Locks were not needed to secure our belongings until seventh grade, when we were first issued combination locks for our gym lockers. We were using lockers that were in changing rooms that also served people from other neighboring towns. I don't think that those locks were truly needed, but it was an exciting new thing for a twelve-year-old. We all signed for our locks, and assured the coach that we understood the responsibility associated with them. Our combinations were written out according to the code that corresponded with the master list. At once we went to work practicing our specific combinations. Some picked up the process quickly; some struggled and needed the assistance of a teammate. Some of us could unlock our locks if we were reading the combination. Some remembered their combination, but couldn't seem to get the exact feel for the lock. The number said one clockwise turn to 4, but you had to feel the mechanics of the lock because it might be a degree past 4. At the very least it was a process, a process of trial and error. I don't remember anyone giving up on the process. I have always struggled with remembering numbers. I kept the little slip of paper with me as a crutch for a long time. In a short period of time we were all locking and unlocking our gym lockers using the combination locks issued to us on that special day.

You may be wondering, "What do a twelve-year-old and a combination lock have to do with my weight issues?" Explore this thought with me. Through the years I have tried programs, products, foods, exercise, and suggestions that helped some-what, but were not the long-term solution that I had sought. They were all part of my combination to unlock a healthy weight. Many of these solutions remain a part of my lifestyle to this day.

Some of the things I tried were not at all beneficial. They were not part of my combination. When we received our locks in seventh grade, some of our numbers were the same numerals that were on our friends' combinations, and some were different. Some of us had the exact same numbers but in a different order. All the locks looked the same, yet each was unique. They were as different as we were. Now do you understand where we're going?

Unique Combinations

Remember: you may be similar to those around you, but you are unique and different, just like your fingerprints. Those who have allowed me to assist them are finding their combinations to a healthy weight. At this writing, I have been set free from my bondage of obesity. I have had the privilege to share in others' searches for their combinations as well. The good news is, it can be done. You can find your combination to a healthy weight and be free from obesity. It's not a miracle pill; there's no magic bullet. There simply is a combination that is right for you.

I know this sounds like a lot of work. I won't tell you it will be a walk in the park. I *will* tell you that it will be worth it. When I speak to groups, my message is always the same: "There is freedom from obesity. May I help you find it?" To get to know my group, this is my opening routine. I ask everyone who has ever struggled with weight to stand. If their struggle just started in the last six months, I ask them to sit down. Most remain standing. Then, like an auctioneer, I start counting up. If you have struggled for one year or less, please sit down. If your struggle has lasted five or less years, please sit down. The drill continues: ten years, twenty years, thirty years, forty, fifty, sixty, seventy years, and people are still standing. Slowly, they see my point revealed before their eyes: If what we were doing actually worked, none of us would still be struggling. Each time I do this little experiment I am amazed at the number of people who have struggled for decades.

Some questions to consider: How long have you struggled? Is dealing with your health consequences easy? How costly is your bondage of obesity? What have you missed out on because you're carrying extra weight? Isn't being overweight a burden?

To me, the burden of having been overweight for forty years was a lot of work. If I have to work at something, I might as well work for freedom instead of struggling in bondage. I am here to tell you that it's worth it! *You are worth it!*

To say I am passionate about this is an understatement. I have spent my whole adult life trying to find exactly the right combination for me. The problem was I was looking for the correct magic bullet for me. Through struggle I have found my combination and have found some basic principles that are included in most of our combinations. This discovery of basic principles has been a blessing to many others as well. Remember: everyone's problem of being overweight looks the same — just like our locks looked the same. The basic principles are the same, just like the same numerals that were available on the locks. Unfortunately, there is no master codebook to consult to find out our combination, but there are some ways to feel the process, just like we had to learn the uniqueness of our individual locks to see if just moving just a degree off the specified number might open the lock. The factor that was so useful in the seventh grade is available to you now, and that is teammates who are working on the combination with you. You also have a coach available. I don't have all the answers, but I have some very good ideas. Working together, we can find your correct answer!

We know the consequences of overweight / obesity all too well. We are touched by the problems associated with this bondage on a very personal level. My concern is that if we don't change the direction and build some momentum in the opposite direction, we are heading for major devastation. Wouldn't you agree that what we are doing is not working?

A New Look?

Has the time come for you to find your combination to unlock a healthy weight? Maybe you have just been given a new lock. Each year we turned in our combination locks at the end of the season. Some years we would get our old lock back, so remembering the familiar combination wasn't difficult. Some years we would receive an entirely different lock. The combination was new, but it wasn't hard to look at our little combination sheet and learn the new sequence of numbers. It was so much easier than the first time, because we knew the basic principle by heart.

Life sometimes gives us new locks. We are going strong, and something happens that changes our combination. I coach people from all stages and situations in life. We have people for whom the issue of weight is a new challenge. Take, for instance, the women who have found themselves entering the change of menopause. Healthy weight was never an issue for them, and suddenly they have added weight in their midsection. They have no idea how it got there or how to get rid of it. Life has just issued them a new combination lock.

Traumatic events have a way of presenting us with new locks as well. Dealing with loss of income or the loss of a home puts our bodies into a realm of new circumstances. I often see stress as a factor that alters our combinations and adds unhealthy weight to the issue. The good news is there are others who have been in your shoes. Their combination is not identical to yours, but with teamwork you can figure out the sequence. Just as our team pulled together when we were first issued our locks, there is an answer for you, within you, and around you.

At least 70 percent of us have not found our correct combination. Can we agree that what we have tried isn't working? As the saying goes: "If you always do what you've always done, you will always get what you have always got!" It has also been said that insanity is doing the same things over and over and expecting different results. I know that was the cycle I was caught in. I thought diet and exercise was the key, and that the problem must be me. I was flawed and destined to be overweight and unhealthy.

Other people weren't struggling. They could eat anything they wanted and stay thin. Well, I was wrong — I was not the problem; I just didn't know the basic principles of living a healthy life. I had bought into the myth of the magic bullet, the one solution. I didn't know better, so I couldn't do better. I'm happy now that I have for the time being found my correct combination for a healthy weight. I'm also aware that I could be issued a brand-new combination lock at any time. I'm also confident that when that time comes and life changes, I will be prepared.

I know the basic principle of unlocking a healthy weight. I have surrounded myself with a team that knows how to unlock healthy weight combinations. They might even have some extra tools that are not in my toolbox just now. I am prepared to ask for help from a master coach who has more experience than I have. The true freedom from obesity is that I have a plan and the confidence to carry out the plan to accomplish positive results.

Combination of Habits

It has been rewarding to watch others take this journey. In this book I will introduce you to a few of them. The exciting thing is that each of them is unique, yet the basic principles are the same. Some found their combinations quickly; some needed assistance from their coaches and teammates, and some had to use a crutch until they were confident in the process. All of those who stayed the course and didn't throw in the towel found their combinations to a healthy weight, and now that they have unlocked their combination once they can consistently unlock it again and again. Even when life issues us another lock, we are prepared to find the new combination. Just like learning anything new, it gets easier with practice.

Have you ever driven to the store and not remembered driving there? When we do something repeatedly, our minds can guide our habits unconsciously. When we have been at an unhealthy weight for as many as seventy-plus years, we have developed habits that support that unhealthy weight. Even unconsciously, we are supporting this condition. That is why we must find our combination and practice it consistently to change the pattern. When we have strongly imprinted unhealthy habits into our brains, it takes work to establish new habits.

As a teenager, once I had learned the combination to my lock in the gym, I could soon unlock my lock while involved in all the locker room conversation. I had unlocked it so many times my hands would just dial the combination without my even thinking about the numbers. My experience with a healthy lifestyle is similar: It now happens unconsciously. I don't think about every bite I take, I don't force myself to go to the gym, and I don't feel deprived. I have found my combination, and I live life! It is a freedom that I don't even think I can express — it is an experience you have to live.

When I am showing others a photo illustrating my heaviest and unhealthiest body, I realize I cannot recreate that body; it would take too much work. Each of us has a combination of habits, you see, whether positive or negative. The blend of habits I had for so many years created obesity, and locked me into the bondage of an unhealthy body. I would have to work hard to recreate those habits and thus recreate the unhealthy body I once had.

I am too happy with my life to work toward that bondage again. New, healthy habits are becoming unconscious habits and are developing into an amazing lifestyle. Throughout this process, I have learned that there are more combinations for me to find. Now that I am free from obesity, I see a greater opportunity for abundant health and bigger rewards. For the first time in my life I love to play. I love going to the gym and running. It thrills me to do things freely that I once forced myself to do because I knew I should. Exercise is so much more fun when it's enjoyment than when it's a requirement.

I tell the students in my classes that through their thoughts and their habits they created the bodies in which they are sitting. People don't like to hear that they created their own problems. Nonetheless, our habits are the combinations we are using. Actually, it works this way with about everything in life. If we are happy, we are choosing habits that support our happiness. If we are sad, we are choosing the habits that support our sadness. My students truly want to achieve a healthy weight, but they struggle to find the answer for themselves.

As I have said, there is not just one answer. It takes a combination of habits that are unique to you. The main problem is that everyone has a solution to offer. They want to present you with this miracle food, this workout plan, this weight loss program, this pill, or this surgery. It might be true that a special food is part of your combination, but be cautious of emphasizing one solution. There are going to be some things that carry more weight than others (pardon the pun). Looking at my personal combination, my lifestyle, some key factors changed my situation from unhealthy to healthy. It is imperative to change our thoughts and our habits if we want to be free from obesity or any other problem in our lives.

The thing I soon realized once I started helping those who wanted help was that they didn't know the factors that supported a healthy combination. All they knew was the advertised solutions that promised to be their magical quick fix. They were in a world of confusion. Many were ready to give up. My first goal was to assure them that help was available and freedom could be achieved.

I am so thankful to have found my combination, and I'm happy to help others in the journey. It is worth it — *we* are worth it. When we know better, we can do better. Most of us don't know better, so we can't yet do better. For a variety of reasons, not everyone will find their combinations. That is very much all right. I wish to support those who want to do better. Always remember: when we know better, we can do better. It is so important to learn a better way. I can help you know better, so that you can do better.

Many years ago, when I turned the little knob to the correct numbers in the correct sequence, the lock would open every time. If I missed one step or turned it in the wrong direction, the lock would not open no matter how hard I pulled. People question me about our program's success rate. I smile and confidently say, "one hundred percent!" They look at me like I'm crazy. Maybe I am. If so, I'll be content with crazy. If you are able to learn the basics, find your combination, and apply it with consistency, healthy weight and freedom from obesity is yours.

The combinations of habits you have now are presenting themselves 100 percent. It is 100 percent of what you don't want, but it's the best you can do. We reap what we sow. It's like the law of gravity, a law that we understand: if you step off a roof you will fall. If you have habits that support obesity, you'll be obese. If you have habits that support health, you'll be healthy.

I also realize that it's hard to break the unhealthy habits of many years' duration. Some people would rather suffer the consequences associated with obesity than change those habits. I acknowledge and respect that, and I ask you this: If you are not content with your health, are you ready to find your combination? The great news is that *you get to choose.* My mission is to share what I know so that those searching can, in time, find their combinations to a healthier weight. It is wonderful to be free from obesity.

Chapter 3

Behold the Pattern

The best way to help people is by developing a relationship with them. The best doctors sit down and get to know their patients. The best teachers have taken the time to understand their students' thought processes. People who provide the best service recognize the needs of their customers. Then they meet those needs to the best of their ability.

Marriages that last decades are founded on a true connection of unconditional love. Having a relationship is a fundamental component to facilitate a positive change. The only way I know to accomplish this is to share my story with you. It is a story of triumph over trial, a story of uncovering the Karen who was hidden and now has found freedom. Someday, I hope you will share your story of triumph over trial with me. Today, ours will be a one-sided relationship. All this is in hope that you will be inspired to make positive changes and then encourage others to continue the cycle.

I am Karen Denise Warren Locklear. I am not the same

person you would have met ten years ago. The woman writing this book is now extremely happy to be free from obesity. That sounds simple and perhaps a little silly, but if you are reading this while you are trapped in an obese body, you may know exactly where I'm coming from. It would be interesting to watch an interview of people who knew me as I was growing up. They would share their perceptions of a totally different person than you are getting to know through this book. It is crucial for you to know some of my history so you can see how your history plays a part in your obesity.

We have already established that freedom from obesity will require a combination of things, not all of them physical. This was a big WOW! for me as I was finding my way. We are not just physical beings. We are a combination of emotional, mental, and spiritual beings as well. Most of the information we have been bombarded with is only about our physical aspect. That is only a small part of the reason we are frustrated and can't seem to change our weight however hard we try. That's why I was compelled to write this book. I would be very selfish to have been set free but not do everything within my power to help as many others as possible.

What are my qualifications? Here is what's on my business card: Karen Warren Locklear, BS, MRS, MM, Ph.T., GRAN-Health Resourceologist. Let me explain my credentials. The BS is in home economics education from Oklahoma State University. I used this degree by teaching in the public schools for sixteen years. I taught in three states. I substituted for all ages, K–12. I taught two years of Life Skills at Kayenta Middle School in Arizona. Most of my teaching experience was at Hollis High School in Oklahoma where I taught Family and Consumer Sciences. I finished my public teaching career in Bonner Springs,

Kansas where I spent two years teaching Kindergarten. In 1989, I received accreditation for my MRS and MM degrees simultaneously. The Master of Resource Services and the Master of Motherhood degrees were on-the-job training and by the seat of my pants.

The year I married my wonderful husband, Ben, I also had the privilege of adopting my fourteen-year-old son, Benji, and my ten-year-old daughter Jenny. Now you understand "on-the-job training and by the seat of my pants." I was only twenty-four at the time. Looking back, it's good to know that love may not be blind, but it's definitely a little naïve. I'm so thankful for these degrees. Ten years later, I took a refresher course for my MM degree when Ben and I adopted our eight-year-old foster daughter Ilia.

In 2002, I successfully completed my Ph.T. — Putting Hubby Through. Of our first thirteen years of marriage, nine were spent supporting and encouraging my husband as he was working hard to achieve his doctorate in Chiropractic. When he was carrying thirty-plus hours a trimester in chiropractic school, I was working three jobs to make ends meet. Keep in mind that every day I was getting continuous education for my MRS and MM degrees. I can assure you it was all worth it.

My final degree was the easiest to get and the most rewarding. It is my GRAN degree. I have been blessed with four wonderful grandchildren: Matthew, Sierra, Kolby, and Chloe. Great pleasure comes from seeing my children grow and develop as parents. They are wonderful parents, and are supported by Brandee, David, and John, their fantastic spouses.

I have titled myself a Wellness Resourceologist. I feel that all of us are resourceologists of one sort or another. You'll soon see how all these degrees connect with my obesity. Don't jump ahead, now — I'm not blaming my obesity on anyone or anything. I'll show you how our relationships with things and our reactions to them contribute to obesity.

Even though we don't have any official, prestigious degrees, we all do things daily that impact the lives of others. The people I have been privileged to work with on their weight issues are amazing. They are masters of caring for others, some to the point of sacrificing self. I'm aware that of the degrees listed on my card only one is official, but even though no accreditation group recognizes the other credentials, they are well deserved. I worked hard for all of them. I continue to hone my skills in daily life. Without knowing your name, I am confident that you understand and have your own list of credentials.

We Give, Give, Give

Hopefully, you now know that we are more alike than different. As I get older, I start to realize the wisdom in this. We tend to feel isolated and see our struggles as our own. Also, we fail to recognize our achievements and focus instead on our limitations. This too plays a part in obesity. Remember, we are not just physical bodies. The people who are most abundant in my classes are mothers. They give, give, and give; they take care of everyone else while sacrificing themselves. Does this describe you? Have you forgotten who you are and become just a caregiver for others? Yes, we are supposed to take care of our families. Yes, we are called to be servants, but if we have sacrificed ourselves, what do we have remaining to give?

I often must remind my students that if they are all used up and totally spent, they will have nothing to give to their families. This is a huge issue for mothers, teachers, nurses, and other caregivers. They give, give, give and go, go, go while forgetting to replenish themselves. They are often overfed yet undernourished. They opt for the quick meal of convenience and sacrifice nutrition. They are caught in a trap that is all too common in today's fast-paced world. This lifestyle rapidly takes its toll. I speak from experience. Remember the credentials I have already shared? I understand busy. I understand what it takes to raise a family today. Even with me working three jobs, we lived below poverty level while Ben was in chiropractic college.

This was the time my weight got totally out of control. We existed on fast convenience food. I drank more soda pop than should be legal. Actually, caffeine was my drug of choice. I didn't realize it at the time, as I was just trying to make it through the day. I rarely drank water. My body was pushed to the max, and I survived on the short-term energy provided by sugar-laden processed foods and the caffeine from soda pop. When I found time on the weekends, I would crash. Everything I did was accomplished out of pure desire to keep going. I was a self-sacrificing wife and mother caught up in this common cycle. I never complained, because that's what I was expected to do, right? This was nothing new; it was what my mom and both my grandmothers had done — give all and sacrifice self. I didn't know better, so I couldn't do better.

I now know there's a better way. In class, it's imperative to remind my students of the guidance the flight attendants give on airplanes: "Mothers, if the oxygen masks deploy, secure your mask first and then assist your children."

This is a vital principle. If we as caregivers become sick or can't function, who will take care of those we are caring for? If we don't learn how to properly nourish and care for ourselves, how can we change? Who is going to be an example of a better way for our children? Is this part of the overweight/obesity problem? I think so. Here is a shocking statistic for you: Today's generation of children is expected to be the first in history not to outlive their parents. The statistic isn't saying they will die at a younger age than their parents, but that their parents will bury them. We already see a steady increase in childhood obesity. How many children do you know who have been diagnosed with type-2 diabetes? How many children do you know who suffer from high blood pressure, a disease that was once seen only in adults? Do I have your attention yet? Is this fast-paced life of convenience worth it? Not only do we need to take care of ourselves in order to be around to take care of others, but we also need to model the behavior.

Stop the Pattern

We neglect the basics to keep pace in this modern world, and we are reaping the consequences. Many of today's diseases are illnesses of modern convenience. I have experienced this personally, and it is one of the reasons I wrote this book for you. I've watched too many families suffer due to this cycle. It has been a pattern in my family for three generations. My goal is to stop the pattern. I am fully aware that I don't make the decisions for anyone but myself, and I am thankful for this. What I can do is change my life by incorporating better decisions that I bring about by renewing my way of thinking. I can also model a healthier lifestyle. We desperately need to see a better way, and we need the support of others who are also making these lifestyle changes. This is a major reason why I teach lifestyle changes based on critical information.

Our students in TLC Lean are changing their lives. They are learning to know better so they can do better. They also benefit from a support group with the same goals. We now watch people regain health and break free from many health consequences associated with obesity in just three months.

My goal is to encourage you. We all know the price of obesity; we are all personally acquainted with this situation. With a few basics and some baby steps it's possible to make incredible changes. Applied consistently, these baby steps can become milestones. As we live and model a healthier, more balanced lifestyle, we have an opportunity to change our family legacy. It is rewarding to see this happening in my family. My daughter, Jenny, is doing a great job finding balance in a fast-paced world. Her children are benefiting from healthier habits. She actually is able to keep up with the busy pace, but unlike my history, she has the health to enjoy her family activities.

I was so out of balance that I was just doing what I needed to do. I was missing out on life. Most of the time, I was doing what was expected, and had to push myself because I wasn't healthy. I was a captive in my own body. Life was something I did, not something I lived. How did this happen? When did it start? Now that I have uncovered the Karen who was buried beneath seventy-five pounds of fat, I think I've found some of the answers. I will share my discovery because I know these answers are not unique to me. Remember, even though we are unique, we are more alike than different. As I reveal my personal discoveries, I encourage you to keep an open mind and heart. You will uncover some beneficial information for your own use.

More than Physical

It's important for us all to understand that we are not just physical in nature. We experience life mentally, emotionally, and spiritually as well, and all these elements affect each other. Let me give you an example. When our students come for a meeting they can check their sugar levels as one of the markers to monitor their progress. At times some of them are alarmed that their sugar has risen. They feel frustrated because they know they did very well all week. They stuck to the plan, so this rise is a shock to them. This becomes a good teachable moment. Physically, they had done everything correctly. I ask them if it was a stressful day, or even better, I tell them it was a stressful day and they will agree. Their bodies were reacting physically to the emotional insult; their hormonal systems were reacting to the stress. It really doesn't matter what type of stress — basically, their bodies were in protection mode.

Here is a jewel of information for you. Our bodies are amazing, and they want to be in balance and healthy. When we don't take care of our bodies, the disease states often are just the body trying to stay in balance and keep us alive. Let's look at my life starting twenty years ago — a working mother with an instant family, who was learning to be a wife while doing her best to raise two teenagers. Stressful? Believe it! Was it worth it? Absolutely! Looking back, would I change anything? Yes. I wouldn't change the experiences, but I would change how I dealt with the experiences. I would heed the advice I have already given you. Caring for myself would be top priority.

Now, when I take care of myself, I have so much more to give. It's a win-win situation. Twenty years ago I would have viewed this as selfish. Now I know that properly caring for my body, mind, and spirit is critical. When this takes precedence, there's more for me to give, and the giving is a pleasure instead of a reaction to an expectation. My motivation completely changed. Do you remember me saying, "I love going to the gym"? When I started to become healthier and more balanced, the joy of living returned. The playfulness returned. Before, most of the things I was doing were getting done, but now they were getting done more efficiently and effectively. Life was worth living. I was not just going through the motions. I was living life!

Chapter 4

Uncovering Karen

Looking back, the puzzle pieces are coming together. The exciting thing for me is to know that we can always improve our lives. For much of my life I was in a routine of what was always done. Most of what I did was similar to the pattern modeled by my mother. In following her example I created many of the same problems. I was not healthy, because just like my mother everyone else took priority. The good news for us is the pattern is being broken. Mom and I are now taking care of ourselves. Are we perfect? Absolutely not! Do we step back into our old ways of thinking and behavior from time to time? You bet! Do we like the way we are living our lives now? Without a doubt. It's worth it! We are worth it! Those we love are worth it!

How I Became Lost

Earlier, I asked, "How did this happen? When did it start?" A year ago the answer was unavailable to me. Now I have some new insight to share. Each day it seems that I am experiencing more joy in life. Looking back I can see how I became lost. In essence, I spent many years buried in my own body. This has been an amazing discovery for me, and this understanding has been a large part of my finding freedom from obesity. Your story will be different, but I'm sure you have a story.

The very young Karen was a slender, bubbly girl. She was fearless and could do anything. She loved to help. "Me do it" was her favorite response, quickly followed by action. This was how I expressed myself for the first five years of life. Things started to happen that changed my world. I saw the struggle of my young parents. My dad lost his arm in a farming accident. I nearly drowned. These events changed how I saw life. Fear was introduced, and I began to realize that I couldn't do everything. I became more timid and not so quick to act. I realize that life happens to all of us, and we must learn to deal with these things as we mature. What I hope you are able to see is how such events and how we perceive them can impact us physically as well as emotionally.

The two critical events that were instrumental in my body changing to carry extra weight happened when I was around five. Just a few months after I turned five, my appendix had to be removed. The trauma was being held down and watching the ether mask coming toward me so they could begin surgery. Part of me shut down that day. I experienced great fear. Today, forty years later, this event is still very vivid in my mind. The emotions associated with that image are still very alive within my heart. That event altered how I perceived life. The very bubbly girl who could do anything without fear started to hide that day.

The other event actually happened prior to this one. A few young families were having a party. A bunch of friends and I were floating around in a backyard pool. The adults were visiting beside the pool while we kids swam. I was four, and had not yet learned to swim. I was floating in a kid-sized blowup inner tube. I slipped through the tube and started to sink. I could see legs and feet kicking above me. I remember trying to grab something, but I was paralyzed with fear. Again, these pictures remain vivid today. One of my parents' friends jumped in and pulled me up. That affected me more profoundly than one might think. Subconsciously, I began to go within myself for protection. Through the years the layers of protection thickened. The world was not the safe place I had always thought it. I needed protection. My body physically changed. I started to put on weight.

Physically, the layers of protection were layers of fat. These came on slowly over the years. Until I was literally uncovered by shedding the excess weight, this connection wasn't even a consideration. Throughout the years, other, less distinct things happened. Little by little I buried myself in a fat fortress. The bubbly little girl was well hidden. A reserved, take-no-chances girl and young lady was who people were allowed to see and know. Nonetheless, I was a happy and functional person. I did anything I wanted. I did everything that was expected. The problem was that with all the insulating fat, very few people really got to know me. By the time my internal energy reached the surface it was dull and muted.

Heart Vision

Here is an observation I made one day that helped me to clarify my mission. Keep in mind that my extended family knew me very well when I was young. We were a close family. They knew the bubbly little girl, who was a tiny thing who sold them hugs and kisses. Last year, since shedding the last forty-five pounds, I ran into one of my cousins at a restaurant. He asked what I was doing. I told him about our weight success program. He already knew that my mom had shed a lot of weight. I told him that since shedding the extra weight I was on a mission to help others break free from their bondage of obesity. He looked at me, puzzled, and said, "I didn't think you ever had a weight problem." I was touched. He had seen my heart! He knew ME! He was looking at me from his heart and never saw the extra seventy-five pounds I once carried on for protection. For forty years he saw the little Karen. This was a *huge* piece of the combination!

Prior to this I had already discovered the power of what I call *heart vision.* All my life my mother struggled with her weight. I want you to understand heart vision in greater detail. Although my mom carried over a hundred extra pounds with her, I knew her heart. My head knew that she was very obese; my head knew that most of her health problems arose from her obesity, but I didn't see these things when I thought about Mom. I saw her heart. Now that she has shed ninety pounds, she's revealing the mom I've always known. I love to see her. It gives me great joy to introduce Mom to the world. The world was missing out. Words cannot fully express the joy I feel to be a part of my mom's transformation. Looking back at old photos is amazing. That 250-pound woman was not the woman I saw. The 160-pound spitfire was the mom I always knew with my heart.

Do you understand now that our weight issues are not just physical? Are you seeing how just using physical solutions might be limiting? I hope you're seeing a much bigger picture, that a new realization is being revealed to you. Do you see that we are more alike than different? Do you understand how your story might be a factor contributing to you weight? I am sharing my heart with you. You can see my heart. It would be the same heart whether it was in my former obese body or in my new lean body. That is why I'm writing this book. My mission is to uncover hearts by helping others shed pounds and inches. For this to happen I must pour out my heart to you. Are you ready for more?

The Emotional and Physical Connection

Recently, while speaking with a doctor, I shared my discovery about my weight being a mode of protection. The doctor made a comment that helped me see another way in which I needed my fat. Unconsciously, I needed it to float. WOW! What he said was true. The fear created by my near drowning had caused an unconscious response within my body. Physically, it created its own flotation device. If I could float, I would not drown, and that fear would be assuaged. It would no longer be needed. I could survive. Now, I love to swim, and I've always been proud that I could float in any position. The last time I went swimming was in my lean body, and I had a hard time floating, but there was no fear. I can swim. I no longer need my personal flotation device. It was free to go. I believe this was a part of my combination. This is also why I believe that as long as we try to shed only the physical weight our success might be limited.

Emotionally, I needed to release the fear and see the world differently before I could release the years of protection. For forty years my covering got thicker and thicker. The solutions I tried for decades were limited. The emotional component was crucial. We must always keep in mind that we are not only physical in nature. Had my obesity been just a physical issue I would have been free many years ago. After, all, I was doing many things correctly to deal with the weight, but these were all physical actions.

When talking about weight issues, I often hear, "I know how to do it. I just need to eat less and exercise more." Truthfully, when I hear that, I want to scream. I lived that eat less and exercise more and *it didn't work!* I lived most of my life on 1,000 to 1,200 calories a day. I always pushed myself to exercise. In 2006, I was faithfully getting up at 4:30 every morning to walk five miles. I did this in a little over an hour, so I was not strolling. I would also do an isometric exercise routine, lift weights, and spend thirty minutes in a far infrared sauna. This was my consistent routine for a full year. I could count the days I missed and they were not many. When I put my mind to something, I'm committed. Lack of willpower has never been an issue. I was also eating very healthily, similar to my present-day diet. Looking at my progress journal, I discovered that despite all that physical effort nothing changed. Did I feel like doing this routine? No, but I thought this was my solution. I thought I just needed to exercise more and eat less. I was wrong. No matter what I did, I weighed 185 lbs. Do you understand why I want to scream when people tell me to exercise more and eat less? It also angers me when people consider the overweight lazy and uncommitted. Shall we all scream together?

This physical solution was not working. If nothing is changing after a year, I thought, why am I killing myself? I stopped getting up at 4:30 a.m., stopped walking, and stopped the isometric and weightlifting routines. I did continue the far infrared sauna, which remains part of my combination today. After stopping all the exercise, what changed? Nothing, absolutely nothing changed. I still weighed 185 lbs. That had become my set point; that was what I weighed.

For twenty-one days I did the master cleanse, which is a process of drinking only a lemon drink made to specific directions. I was faithful. Did I lose weight? Yes, I lost twenty-three pounds. When I started adding fruit juices to gradually get back to the healthy foods I was already eating, every one of those twenty-three pounds returned. I felt great and had an abundance of energy, but my consistent 185-pound body had returned. I was happy; I no longer weighed over 200 pounds. I was wearing mostly size 14 clothes, and if I sucked in I could get into some size 12. This was much better than the 212-pound-plus body I tightly squeezed into a size 18.

The Combinations

One May, I committed to a totally raw food diet. I lived the entire month on raw, living foods. Once again, I was committed and didn't cheat. The experience was wonderful. It included studying Ann Wigmore and her amazing work. My daughter, Ilia, and I spent ten days at the Wigmore Institute learning and living this lifestyle. When the ten days were complete, I felt fine, my skin glowed, and my hair was shiny and healthy.

My walking routine was eight miles a day. One day I had the energy to enjoy walking twelve miles. I felt and looked great and had tons of energy, but didn't lose one pound that entire month. I was staying at 185 pounds.

This frustration with physical solutions was not new. Efforts to make my body healthy and lean had begun many years ago. Mom and my grandmothers were always on a diet. My search for answers and help began in elementary school. A friend and I, together with our moms, joined a gym for women. We drove thirty miles to the gym multiple times a week. This was in addition to the PE classes in school. Most of my life I was on some kind of special eating plan. I knew all the Weight Watchers plans by heart. I'm thankful to Weight Watchers and other such programs. If I hadn't been working on some such plan, there's no telling how heavy and unhealthy I'd have gotten.

About twenty years ago, I reached my goal weight. Weight Watchers was my tool for this success. For two and a half years I worked as a leader. This was essential for keeping the weight off. I knew that without a plan and some accountability the thirty pounds would soon return. Again, I'm thankful for this part of the combination; it taught me the importance of team support and encouragement.

This constant search for a solution, and the struggle to be free, was the boundary that framed my life. I was comfortable in that condition, which had become my normal mode of operating. I did not consider myself limited; I was content in knowing how to function within these parameters. Total freedom from the bondage of obesity was not really a consideration.

My struggle had a purpose. Strength often arises from struggle, and empathy is usually a byproduct of it. In my case, passion was cultivated in struggle. Daily, I see how winning my battle with excess weight is a blessing. Watching the transformation as others discover their combinations to unlock their healthy weight is amazing. To say that finding freedom is easy would be misleading. What I can say with all surety is, it's worth it. *You* are worth it.

Today, I am writing to you as a free woman. The bubbly little girl is back. I am experiencing life again from the perspective of the little Karen, the one whose family has always known my heart. I'm not dull and muted by the fat that for so long was my life preserver. There is no need for me to be shy and reserved. People know me as friendly and happy. They don't consider me conceited and aloof as they once did.

I'm vibrant and energetic. It doesn't take every ounce of energy just to make it through a busy day. I am free from obesity, and enjoying my life not just going through the routine because that's what is expected of me. I can run and play with my grandchildren, and it thrills me to play till they're worn out and I'm still ready for more. Life is much better uncovered. There's no need for self-sacrifice. This is a win-win situation. I can take care of myself, and be an even better wife, mother, and grandmother.

Chapter 5

Just Like Mom

We have already established that freedom from obesity requires a combination of elements. We have a better understanding of the emotional component. Now let's take a look at the mental component. Most of our habits start with a thought. Over time these habits become so common we consider them just a part of who we are.

After years of study in health and nutrition, I've come to realize that many of our health consequences are not genetic — they are habitual. I'm not discounting genetic impact. I am saying that many common family health problems materialize because we are repeating the same habits. One doctor whom we enjoy learning from states, "You didn't inherit bad genes, you inherited bad habits." I agree. Of course this perspective requires that we take more ownership of the problem, but that also gives us more control of the outcome. We might not be able to change our genes, but we can change our habits!

I share no genes with my children. At age eight, Ilia was the youngest when she became part of our family. Many habits are already established by that age, but habits can change quickly. I have also seen that even with no genetic connection you can look at photos of my two adopted daughters and me and swear that they had my genes.

My mother and father are my biological parents, so I share their genes. It would be easy to declare that I had no choice but to be obese, and easy to blame all my health problems on my genetics. The problem with that solution is it's not true. I am no longer obese, and no longer have all the health problems I once accepted as inevitable. At age seventeen, while doing the paperwork in preparation for gall bladder surgery, it was scary to list all my family's health problems. I'm thankful that our health isn't entirely dependent on genetics, and extremely happy to know that we can change our thoughts and habits and override many of the genetic factors.

Let's look at how our thoughts can affect our weight. All my life I wanted to be just like Mom, who has always been my best representation for love. I wanted to grow up to be kind, generous, caring, and loving, just like her. As you mature from childhood into adulthood, you take on characteristics both positive and negative. I have discovered that some of the habits and characteristics I emulated weren't so positive. I am confident that Mom didn't want to have these negative habits and characteristics, and she would rather not have passed them on to me.

In the process of discovering the solution to my health struggles, awareness of some of these instances has been revealed. When I was five I had my appendix removed; then, at seventeen, my gall bladder had to be removed. Because of our family's eating habits, I suffered from acne, obesity, and female health problems, just like Mom, who'd had her appendix removed at age five, her gall bladder removed, and had suffered the same cascade of health problems.

In light of the previous chapter, my mom nearly drowned at a young age as well. Now we know that that has no relationship to our genes. Genetics are a physical aspect. We are not just physical, but mental, emotional and spiritual beings, and they are all interconnected, integrated into our complete personhood. No part can be separated out or overlooked without affecting the others parts. Can we agree that we don't just inherit genes, but also inherit habits and lifestyles?

When I think of the "perfect" mom and grandmother, I think of my mother, Nancy Warren. When I became Mom and Gran, I realized I had become like her. I topped the scales at over 200 pounds just like Mom. I had not only Mom as an example, but both of my grandmothers also weighed over 200 pounds. So much of what we do is habit acquired from the examples modeled for us. Unconsciously, I showed love by doing for others and paying no attention to how it affected me. I showed love by serving quick and easy foods that everyone loved, though these were not necessarily the foods that were best for us. I had become just like Mom.

In our family, love was shown with food. This is not unique to my family. Every time we were going to get together, food was the main subject of interest. I come from a line of good cooks. This probably had an influence on me becoming a home economics teacher. My mother and her mother were both teachers. Do you think I inherited a teaching gene? I think it was their thought and habits that influenced me to become a teacher. If we were to actually take the time to consider our habits, we might be amazed how they formed. Our lifestyles are just combinations of habits. It takes just as much time to form a negative habit as a positive one. All habits, though, begin with thoughts.

There are many influences that affect our thoughts. Family is a very strong influence. If my mother had learned how to create a lean lifestyle before I was born would I have struggled with my weight? There are no simple answers. We are complex and every part of our combination to a healthy weight influences the other parts.

Going to the movies has always brought me pleasure. I love a good movie. As a young child two of the movies I watched were *Cinderella* and *101 Dalmatians.* In those movies, think about the people who were kind and generous. What did they look like?

They were overweight. They were jolly. The evil people were thin, like Cinderella's evil stepmother and the fiendish Cruella DeVil. Do you see how, on an unconscious level, I didn't want to be lean? I wanted to be kind and generous, so I needed to be overweight and jolly. Would you trust a skinny Santa Claus? Right or wrong, on a subconscious level I perceived thin people as mean and evil. This was also reinforced by some of the people in my life. My entire family was jolly. They were very giving and loving — and they were all overweight. As a young child, this was deeply imprinted into my thinking.

Our Combinations

We are not just physical beings. We are a combination of our thoughts, our emotions, and our spirit. This is why I believe that most of our weight-loss programs fail. They do not address the whole person, the basics are not known or practiced, and we do not discover our unique combinations.

It wasn't until I had unlocked my combination to a healthy weight that I even considered my thoughts, emotions, and spirit. For forty years the things I tried fell short, because at my core I didn't want to be lean. That discovery amazed me. It didn't really matter how good the solutions were — until I cleared and nourished my whole person, all physical solutions would fail. The world's healthiest diet and best exercise program would be limited by my own thoughts.

I remember when someone I loved went through a life crisis and lost a lot of weight. When she was heavy she was happy and bubbly; when she was thin she was unhappy and unfriendly. As a young child, I equated her unhappiness with her loss of weight. Do you understand? Is it possible that you have thoughts that limit your progress in finding your combination to a healthy weight? This pattern of thinking is still a challenge today. Even though my mom has shed the weight and knows the healthier habits she should choose, old habits die hard. When company is expected, those old ways want to rise up.

Could your thoughts be limiting your progress?

Chapter 6

Watch Your Language

Every child has been told, "Watch your language." When we hear statements like "Watch your mouth, that's a bad word, good children don't talk like that," or "Don't ever use that word again," we think that the speaker is referring to foul language. When I ask my students to watch their language, I'm not speaking of words that I find offensive. I ask them to reframe their wording because of the power of words. It has nothing to do with how their words affect others, and everything to do with how their words affect them. Offensive words are destructive, and the destructiveness primarily affects the one speaking the words. Those around them are not immune to the harm, especially young children who hear such language, but the greatest damage is to the speakers themselves, because they believe their words, and store them in their minds and hearts.

We all know the power of the tongue. The Bible cites it many times. It is often referred to as a small rudder on a large ship.

The tongue is a small but mighty force. I hope this chapter will give you a new understanding of how our use of words affects our behavior. We've already determined that our minds and hearts play an important role in shedding weight and becoming free from obesity. It is also important for us to realize that we may be unknowingly sabotaging our success. When I visit with our students, I often ask them to speak their thoughts in a different way. It's amazing how things can be transformed just by changing a word here and there. It's a joy to watch students change their lives by making a few changes, often sparked by changing a word.

Precisely which words do I consider offensive and destructive? Well, let's start with one that everyone reading this book has used: This awful word is "diet!" Yes, diet, and here's why diet is a dirty word: Diets don't work. They are depriving and restricting, and they contribute to failure. Diets are impossible to follow. So why do we still diet? It's like trying to pump air into a flat tire that has a hole in it. It just doesn't work. It may seem to take the air for a while, but then the hole wins. Eventually, we just give up, frustrated and exhausted.

What emotions do you feel when you read the word "diet"? I hate the word. The only reason I ever use it is to communicate to those still trapped in this unsuccessful routine. When I was obese, diet and dieting consumed my life. I was always searching for the answer and spent all my time looking for the latest and greatest diet plan, each time hoping it would be the final answer to free me from obesity. It was a never-ending emotional roller coaster of hopes, promises, and devastation. I came into this world a dieter. My mother was a chronic dieter. My language has always included "diet" and all the other limiting words. I thought like a dieter. I had perfected the dieting lifestyle. I was well versed in the language, attitudes, and behavior of dieting.

Let's look at the word "diet." It contains the word "die"! No one wants to die — we want to live! That's why in my communications I use terms like *food plan, eating habits, food choices, life plan,* etc. In some of my papers, I actually put a slash mark through the word "diet" and write "life" above it to make this point. What are we doing to ourselves on a subconscious level when we use this word? My hopes and dreams are to help others off this emotional monster, whatever it takes. I believe it can start by eliminating destructive habits, and this starts by eradicating the word "diet." I live every day not bound by the limits of some diet or restrictive notion of what will help me lose weight. We all want to live and be free of the bondage of obesity. Some amazing transformations could be made if we eliminated the word altogether.

Next on my list of useless words are *loss* and *lose.* Again, these words must occasionally be used to communicate with those trapped on that endless emotional roller coaster. Who really wants to *lose* or report a *loss*? I've never heard anyone at a ballgame say, "Yeah, we came to lose!" I've never heard of anyone celebrating a loss. The only time these words are used this way is in association with weight. Groups of people watching their weight celebrate losing and losses. How does it make us feel when we lose? Isn't a loss usually a time of mourning? Maybe on a deeper level we really don't want to lose or experience a loss. Maybe this is what's causing some of our struggle, and part of the reason we lose weight and then regain it.

Have you ever lost something precious to you? How did you feel? I remember losing a special ring. I searched high and low but didn't find it right away, though I often thought about it and subconsciously kept it in mind. I think we do this when we lose weight: We initially celebrate the loss, but then we find it and put it back on. We have become comfortable at that weight and the habits that created that body. Too often, when we regain the weight it returns with added pounds. In our classes we jokingly say, "It found friends while it was lost, and decided to welcome these extra pounds to our bodies."

At TLC Lean we don't celebrate losses or note how much weight we've lost. We celebrate *wins*. They are numerous and as unique as the individual. We celebrate inches taken up in belts, climbing stairs without thinking, blood pressure normalizing — the list is endless. It thrills me to hear our students discuss their wins before meetings. Words can't express the joy when these Leaners share their wins. What is it worth to Jerry to announce that he can bend down, put on his socks and shoes, and tie his shoes without assistance? It's priceless. We love to hear wins, and we love for the wins to multiply.

To help you lose the habit of using the words "loss" and "lose," let me offer you some more encouraging options. At TLC Lean we *shed* weight, *let go* of pounds and inches, *release* unwanted fat, and *reduce* size. When we let go, shed, and release, we are less likely to try to find what has gone. I often have to remind students in the process that this extra weight is *gone*. I must remind them that this is a permanent situation. Do words play a part in our constant struggle? I think so. I hear and see it with the wonderful people who are making this transition. Do you understand now why it's important to watch your language?

Pay attention to the words you use. You might be surprised at how your language is affecting your results. I hear people say things like: "I'm watching my weight," or "I'm counting my calories." I ask, "What are you watching your weight do? Is it going up and down on that never-ending roller coaster? Why are you counting calories? Does knowing how many you're consuming change anything?" Our wording is important. I don't want our students to just be "weight watchers" and "calorie counters." I want them to be lean and healthy. That's why we call our program TLC Lean. Everyone could use a little tender loving care. *Lean* actually has a double meaning. We want everyone to have a lean, health body, and we want everyone to lean in a different direction. We have leaned in the same direction for years and reaped only poor results. Now it's time to lean another way. We have leaned on man's ways and altered foods to create this mess. Now, let's lean on God's ways and His pure foods to have a healthy and abundant life.

I call my students Leaners. When they come in or I see them in public, I refer to them as "Leaning men" and "Leaning ladies." I ask them, "How are you leaning?" I want them to think lean and live lean. I don't want them stuck in the same vocabulary that has limited their success. Successful people use language that supports their accomplishment.

I also try to curtail any negative language, such as "I can't," "Nothing works," or "I'm so..." We all know the trap this language can be. "I am" and "I have" statements are very powerful and can be harmful. I spend a lot of time redirecting language. When someone says, "I am diabetic" or "I have high blood pressure," I call them by name and say, "You have the symptoms of high blood pressure; you are not the disease, nor should you be limited by it." We often become our diagnosis or our disease. If we use that as a part of our language and believe it, change is hard to make. When you live with a diagnosis for forty-plus years, it can be a hard habit to break. If you get healthy and no longer have the symptoms but still claim the disease, is it more likely to return? I believe so.

Since "I am" statements are so powerful, I recruit that power in my life. I'm very careful how I use these two little words. I have made myself consciously aware of them, and I watch what they produce. In my old body, I would say things like: "I am fat, I am a mess, I am ugly, I am lazy, and I am sick." Once I put my "I am's" in their proper place they began to help me change my life. Now I say things like: "I am lean, I am organized, I am cute, I am active, and I am well." Do you see the contrast? Do you feel the difference? Can you grasp the power of these two tiny words?

Another part of this technique is to make sure our actions support our words. When our students are shedding or releasing the weight, I constantly remind them to use those words. Likewise, I also ask them to get rid of their larger clothes in the process. It's important for them to be reminded that they have let go of the pounds and inches and will no long need those clothes. To some this is a fearful thought. Consider for a moment: If you've been dealing with a weight challenge most of your life, you've been large and small and many sizes in-between. You have a wide range of sizes of clothes grouped in your closet by big, bigger, and biggest instead of by seasons. This has been your pattern for most of your life. You have ridden the emotional roller coaster for fifty or sixty years. Do you see how fearful an experience getting rid of oversized clothing can be, when nothing has ever worked before over the long term?

When I tell them that it is important for them to rid themselves of clothes that no longer fit, I often see terror in their eyes. You would think that I had just pulled their safety net out from beneath the high wire they are balanced on. For decades they have lost and gained. The loss they experienced for many years was eventually found and often multiplied. They were always prepared: They had clothes of every size to meet the needs of their ever-changing bodies. They had made a major investment in these ever-changing bodies. The investment was expensive. They had spent much time, effort, and money on a flexible wardrobe. Letting go of the comfort of having a way back was big. They were being asked to venture into uncharted territory.

Wardrobe Emotions

While we are on the subject of wardrobe, I want to share some thoughts with you. Most of our "stuff" is emotionally charged. We commonly keep possessions because of the emotions attached to them. Clothing is no different. It may be one of the main possessions that call to mind life's special events and memories. I have saved a few special dresses. Fortunately for me they were small sizes. When I reached my healthy weight, I went through the closet and removed all the clothes that no longer fit — everything in the closet! It was an amazing experience. I recorded it on video because it was an emotional event. Keep in mind I always dreamed of having a size-12 closet. It would contain nothing larger than a 12. I thought that this would be the perfect place for me to be. When I finally unlocked my combination to a healthy weight, I didn't own anything in size 12; my largest size was a 10. All my adult life I had thought *if I could just get into a 12 and nothing larger that would be perfect.* This is one of the reasons I ask our Leaners to be open-minded. They often transform into bodies beyond their wildest dreams.

Unloading my closet entailed a wide and varied range of emotions. As I removed each garment to fold and put in the box, a flood of memories was attached. Not everyone will go through this, though for some it could be a deeply emotional experience. That is why language is a factor. Even though we are letting go of the clothes, we can keep the precious memories. Could this be part of the connection with loss? If we see that we have lost weight and are now losing our clothes and the memories associated with them, could this be a hurdle to letting the weight go? It is so important to look at the wins. We still have the memories, and now we have a chance to make even happier memories in leaner bodies. We also need to remember that when we are in healthier bodies, the chances are greater that we will enjoy longer and more productive lives in which to make better memories.

Our oversized clothes can be a marker for success, but they can also be a bridge back to an unhealthy weight. This is why we focus on the win instead of the loss. I wanted to remove any bridge back to my unhealthy body. I wanted to make it more challenging to go back than to move forward. We want everyone set up for success. That is why TLC Lean is a *weight success* program instead of a *weight loss* program. Unfortunately, I have to talk weight loss to reach those looking for help.

It seems to help when Leaners can give away the clothes that are too large for them. It's common for them to give them to other Leaners. Someday we hope to have a way to redistribute these clothes so they can experience the joy of their clothes benefiting others. It's rewarding when they let go, break that pattern, and get rid of the clothes that are too large. It's rewarding to see them tuck in their shirts and wear belts. The men often mark their progress by the notches of their belts. Some get to wear their thirty-year-old belts; some get to buy new belts and even smaller clothes than they've ever worn. It's a lot more fun to shed and reduce than to lose or experience a loss. Don't you agree?

I find it funny that *diet, loss,* and *lose* are all four-letter words. When I introduce people to our program I tell them immediately that I don't like these words, which I feel have the potential to cripple their success. I ask them to remove them from their daily vocabulary. When they hear my thoughts, they understand. I hope that someday these words are never again used in association with our bodies.

I mentioned earlier that my father lost his hand when I was very young, and that I lost my appendix and gall bladder. I still function very well, but a loss is still a loss. The loss of any body part is traumatic. A major loss for me was when I lost the opportunity of having children after having had two ectopic pregnancies. Even though we do not like our weight situation and the resulting health effects, it is part of us. What has been with us a long time becomes part of our body image. Separation from it must be gentle. Could it be traumatic to have it removed surgically? We must be ready to let it go. We must be willing to shed the weight. If we are not ready, and we lose it for others, or are not releasing for the right reasons, it will return. That is why the endless emotional roller coaster is such a popular ride. So let's focus on the wins, the gains, and the benefits of shedding unhealthy weight. Let's model success as we celebrate wins and the long-term benefits of a healthier weight. Let's watch our language. Let's help people off that roller coaster and onto the ride of a lifetime!

Chapter 7

What You Think About, You Bring About

Now we need to consider our thoughts. Yes, let's think about our thoughts. We have already seen that we inherit not just genes, but habits. We also inherit our thoughts and thought patterns. These are passed to us in verbal and non-verbal communications. Positive thinkers tend to raise positive thinkers; negative personalities seem to hang around negative personalities. When we are down, we tend to find others who can commiserate with us.

Now, do we inherit a gene for positive thinking? Do we inherit a gene for negative thinking? I think not. If we don't inherit a thinking gene, we have a great opportunity, because it means we can change our thoughts. We can also employ language to help us with this process, and we can help others to change by using language as a link to new thoughts or a new way of thinking.

The place to start our exploration of thought is to evaluate our present situation. At this time, the body I have and the things I am able to do are created by my pattern of thoughts. The experiences now demonstrated in my life were incubated in my mind before they became a part of my physical body. The body I live in now is very different from my body ten, twenty, or forty years ago. The body I live in now is much improved from my old one. How did this happen? I changed my thoughts! I changed how I view life in general. I changed how I nurture my thoughts to the tiniest detail. This may sound foreign to you. Just a few years ago it was a foreign concept for me as well. It was a gradual discovery, and I would like to reveal it to you. This is something very useful and potentially very powerful. It's a major component in unlocking my combination to a healthy weight, and it can be a potent tool for any aspect of our lives.

Our thoughts are like seeds. They can remain dormant if they aren't cared for. In any given day, innumerable thoughts flit through our minds. Most have nothing to connect with and no place to grow, so they are quickly gone. We also have thoughts that embed deeply because they find common ground or a place to connect. They closely resemble thoughts that are already present and being cared for. They are supported and nourished by our language. We have all heard the saying, "The rich get richer and the poor get poorer." We have seen people who seem to win at everything. No matter what they're doing, it looks like "Lady Luck" is on their side. In my case, I was fat; no matter what I did, I was fat. Did it have anything to do with my thoughts? I think so. I thought of myself as fat, I talked as a fat person would, and my emotions and habits supported my fat body.

Looking back over my lifetime, I was not always fat. I *thought*

I was fat. I used the language of a fat person, and developed the habits of a fat person. My emotions supported these habits. I ate to feel good, I ate when I felt bad, I ate when I had an emotional hole instead of physical hunger. I ate to celebrate, and I ate to commiserate with others. I ate when it was time to eat, even if I wasn't hungry. If someone offered me food or a sweet treat, I ate it. I ate just to be eating. It was an activity I preformed even when I was stuffed to the limit. My thoughts and emotions supported this behavior.

Remember: I was born to an overweight mother who had struggled with her weight most of her life. She watched her parents and many other family members struggle similarly. Did we all inherit "fat genes"? I think not. We inherited "fat thoughts." We helped them spread and take root by using our "fat language," and we nourished them with our "fat emotions." We were trapped in a fat lifestyle. We thought about food, we talked about food, and our emotions were reflected in our food. Food held a central position in our lifestyles. But food was not the problem; *how we thought about food* was the problem, and it was enhanced by our language and tied to our emotions.

When I think of family, I think of food. It is not in any way a negative perception. Actually, it's a very positive one. The best cooks came from my family. No one was ever allowed to leave one of our homes hungry. In fact, if you weren't totally stuffed to the point of misery, the ladies didn't feel they had done a good job. The food was always delicious and of the best quality. At large family gatherings the tables were not set for family members to dine; rather, they overflowed with the best of the best recipes prepared to perfection. The amount of food wasn't calculated to accommodate the number of guests; it was brought according to what each mama wished to share. If she knew that cousin James would be there, and he loved that mama's apple pie, the best apple pie was at the top of the list of things she would bring. We've always had the best family gatherings: The food and fellowship were heavenly, and we'd eat until we couldn't eat another bite. Then we would relax and rest while our bodies attempted to digest the overabundance. We were miserably happy. The leftovers were safely stored, but always easily accessible "just in case" someone got hungry.

Just describing this special time with family makes my mouth water as I think of all the good food. It was all made from scratch using the finest ingredients. Best of all, it was made with love. Everyone has thoughts about food, and those thoughts are just as unique as each individual. They are ideas that were passed from generation to generation, and are deeply imbedded into our culture. Such family gatherings were not exclusive to our family. My description matches gatherings of the families I have been around my whole life. Our experiences are similar and our thoughts are similar. We communicate these thoughts, and solidify them into habitual patterns and lifestyles with the help of our language and emotions.

That is not a bad thing. It's a powerful thing. If we create a lifestyle that's not beneficial, we have the power to change it. It starts with our thoughts. Now that I am free from obesity, I think differently, speak differently, and behave differently. I changed the things that weren't beneficial, but I'll keep the thoughts, language, and habits that are. I still cook and prepare my food with love. I still prepare my very best and think of what others might enjoy. What's different is how I think of the food. Is it healthy? Is it nourishing to the body? Is it fuel instead of tasty filler? Is anyone sensitive or allergic to any of the ingredients? Will it be an unnecessary temptation? Will we feel like playing after the meal? My thoughts have changed for the better, and so have my lifestyle and my health. For things to improve it was necessary for me to change my thoughts. This was a huge component of unlocking my combination to freedom.

In our TLC Lean classes we discuss our thoughts. This is a powerful thing. It's amazing to hear someone say something from his or her heart and then experience an "ah-ha!" moment. We know that change is on the horizon. With the support of positive language and positive emotions, healthier habits can lead to a healthier lifestyle. It is common for thoughts to change in this environment. No matter how good the program or product is, if the thoughts stay the same the success of that program or product will be short-lived. Participants who don't change their thoughts are still stuck on that emotional roller coaster.

One of the first things I tell my Leaners in class is: "The body you are sitting in is your own creation. You created this body by your thoughts, words, and actions, and you supported it with your emotions." An overweight body has become their lifestyle, and if they don't make changes it will be their legacy. That is a hard thing to acknowledge, but in their hearts they know it's true. I don't believe it was their fault. Most people simply don't know better. If we know better, we can do better. You are reading this because you want to know better so you can do better. That's why people become a part of TLC Lean. They want to know better. That's why the tagline in our logo is, LEARN, LEAN, LIVE. We must first learn a different way. We must lean in a different direction. We must live life fully, free from the limitations of our old ways.

Most likely we have been stuck in those old ways for a long

time. Transformation is not often made overnight. I can't really tell you how long it took me. I've been searching for help for most of my life, actively trying to break free for many years. Out of sheer determination I had some success, but it was short-lived until I started to change my thoughts.

Chapter 8

We Came to Win

With anything new, finding a place to start often seems to be a stumbling block. I wonder how many blessings have we missed in life just because we didn't make the first move. Daily, I struggle with where to begin, and this is a continuous battle. We know we need to make changes but truly don't have a clue where to start. You are at this moment looking for information. That's a great place to start. I commend you for investigating your options. Every great journey begins with a first small step. To provide you the information you're seeking, I too must make beginning steps into uncharted territory.

Why don't we start this journey at the beginning? I believe that within every one of us is a mission that is to be fulfilled in this lifetime. We are on this earth because we are winners, and we have a passion to share. Some of us let it unfold gradually, while others dive right in and begin living their mission, or passion, full throttle from the start. Over the years as I watch others, especially my children and grandchildren, I'm reminded of who I am and what I have to offer. Let me emphasize again that we all have greatness within us and we all have something special to offer.

Watch a very young child as he or she starts to navigate this world. Everything is fresh and new and full of possibilities. Do you remember that feeling? Until lately, I had lost all the wonder and sense of discovery. Within the last few years I have being making my way back to that place where true possibility is generated. I was a child ready to share everything. There wasn't anything I couldn't do! I was always looking for someone to help or some way to serve.

My parents said that as soon as I could walk and talk, "Me do it!" was my special slogan, and I followed it up with action. This "Me do it!" attitude was reinforced by positive exchanges. I received smiles, "thank you," "good girl," pats on the back, and other expressions of gratitude. I soon found out that one type of exchange was money. I not only received the wonderful words and acts, but was also given cash sometimes. Wow! Money was a little different. It was something I could hold on to and something I could measure. Eventually I realized it could also be exchanged for things I wanted.

I was now in business. I still loved the words and pats, but I greatly enjoyed the nickels and dimes. Sometimes quarters and half-dollars rewarded my service. This evolved into a good little enterprise. Before long I was exchanging hugs and kisses — complete with a snaggle-toothed smile — for money. I loved to feel and count the money. I kept it in a pink, three-foot-tall bank that had the three famous monkeys: hear no evil, see no evil, speak no evil. It was a huge project for me to fill this special bank. I wanted to fill it, and I knew that I couldn't take out any of my precious money and still fill the bank.

The emotions and energy that return as I reminisce is amazing! We all have our stories that have positive emotions and energy attached. I was blessed to have them from the very beginning, as I was born to a very loving and caring couple who supported me with every fiber of their being. My lessons in exchange were never one sided. I didn't always get money, nor did I always get a thank-you. The giving fueled me; the getting was a bonus. Another lesson was that the more things I did for others the greater the possibility of reward. This is not unique to me. My children and grandchildren have learned these lessons as well, and quickly learn whom they want to serve and share with. When there's never a smile or a thank-you, desire to serve that person wanes. We soon learn that good hugs and kisses come from Mom and Dad, while grandparents are often "the big spenders." Aunts and uncles were supportive of my little enterprise. It was a great little cash machine. It was portable and went everywhere I did. Family was my clientele. My cousins enjoyed giving me pennies, nickels, and dimes for hugs and kisses. We all found benefit in the exchange. Not everyone wanted a hug or a kiss, nor did I want to hug or kiss everyone. Mine was a special service, and I learned when and where it was needed.

Are you wondering why I'm sharing this with you? It's because we all have special gifts to offer and services to share. Just as each of us has a unique mission, I believe we deserve to be rewarded with an exchange for our services. That exchange can come packaged in many ways. You can't beat seeing people light up when you've shared part of yourself with them. My mission is to light up lives by helping people uncover their hearts.

How could I help someone in that way? I just described to you how I was happy to serve and share while reaping the rewards and benefits of making exchanges with others, mostly family. At around five years of age that began to change somehow: that blissful little girl was lost and became fearful. In response to some events that impacted me, I began to withdraw into myself. I no longer saw everything as fresh and full of possibilities. I became shy and didn't want to try new things. Life seemed a struggle. The world wasn't as friendly, and I had to protect myself. Mom and Dad were still very supportive, and all of my grandparents had more confidence in me than I had. There were many things I did well. I was a high achiever and was kind and caring of others, but my motivation wasn't the same. Most of what I now did was out of obligation and because it was expected. The joy and love of doing had gone.

I began to change physically as well. I no longer felt pretty. I started to get pudgy, and everything I did required more energy. My light was there, but by the time it got through all the stuff I had surrounded myself with it wasn't very bright. My family could still see my light! They knew my heart. I was content, and from all evidence, everything was fine; everything was normal. I fit in with the real world. The problem was, deep down in my heart and soul I knew there had to be more, but during that period I was too involved in my life to see it.

Many people become so involved in life that they lose sight of their mission. Remember: we are all winners and we all have something special to offer. My father, for example, is an excellent farmer. He loves farming, and it is truly his passion. Other farmers seek his advice. Dad plowed his first field when he was eight years old. He really wanted to farm, and he has never lost his focus on farming. That's what makes him truly successful. Many people hold to their life's mission, which in turn supports their lives. In some ways, we are all entrepreneurs, and if we hold fast to our mission it will support us in life.

My desire to help people has always been strong. I love to teach and I'm good at it. I've been teaching all my life, but it wasn't until I got back to my mission that the passion returned. We should take advantage of every opportunity to learn and apply these lessons to our lives.

For the past several years my husband, Dr. Ben Locklear, and I have been on a journey to improve our health. I'll share our journey with you in hopes that you can apply what we've learned to your own life and help strengthen your mission. Ben and I have learned many things and have watched our health improve enormously. We have discovered that although we might want a quick fix, or something to add to what we are currently doing, health is a lifelong journey, not a destination; we will always be in a struggle. We have learned on this journey that no matter how well we feel, look, or believe our level of health to be, there is always a higher level.

Springboard to Another Level

When you are just beginning to play a sport, basketball, for example, you must first learn the fundamentals. Then you can start playing in elementary games. In a few years, as your skills develop, you might play on junior and senior high school teams. If you choose to work on your skills — let me repeat that — if you choose to work on your skills, you mighty progress to college or professional basketball. Even pro basketball players are always trying to improve their game. In contrast there are many, actually the majority, who never move beyond the fundamentals. The great news in all of this is that we get to choose! We choose our progress by the commitment we make and the continuous actions we take. I played high school basketball. I loved being on the team. I even liked sitting on the bench and supporting the team during our games. My enjoyment arose from practicing and traveling with the team. I really didn't care for the stress of being on the court and feeling pressured to make all the right moves, so I was content to play from time to time when my mistakes weren't critical for the team. That's the level of participation I chose.

That's what we do with our health as well. Ben and I have often discussed such questions as "What is health? How do we decide if we are healthy? Why are some people always struggling with illness, while some seem to never get sick?" We believe we have insight into this matter, as we've consistently worked to improve our health through education and application.

What is health? The answers are as different as each individual. Some people are healthy if they're able to wake up and breathe somewhat freely. Some are healthy if they can make it to their favorite chair and lift the remote to enjoy a day of TV. Some are healthy if they can live a busy lifestyle with caffeine and sugar to keep them going. Some are healthy if they can work and play hard, use no chemical stimulants, and avoid illness. Some are healthy when they live an active life free from physical limitations. Some are happy to be in their eighties or nineties, doing anything they please, which often includes caring for those who are younger and sicker. Just like basketball, there are many levels to health, and the individual determines these levels. Each person gets to choose what level of health he or she wants to achieve. If an individual is content at a particular level, there's no need to make changes and move to a different one. An individual who is not content, however, becomes uncomfortable to the point that he or she makes changes. Most often those changes are prompted by a health crisis — an illness, a diagnosis of a disease, or the loss of ability to do something we could do before. Whatever the case, a tipping point has been reached and changes can now begin. Often such changes must come with education, so the individual can determine the options and formulate a plan.

As long as we are comfortable and happy where we are, no changes are needed. Unfortunately, I think that's exactly where most people are with regard to their health. That is where Ben and I were seven years ago. I was a 212-pound woman with awful menstrual cycles, adult acne, infertility, thinning hair, fatigue, and depression. I was healthy. Because of upper cervical care, my horrible allergies and asthma were gone. I couldn't grow healthy hair or nails or carry a pregnancy, but I was healthy. In our clinic we would watch "healthy people" struggle and not get the pain relief and sustained health we knew they deserved. This prompted us to start seeking answers to help our patients achieve better health. This need became our tipping point. We realized that we didn't have to be content where we were, and could move our health to another level.

That is how we have changed our lives. We have spent several years dedicated to knowing better so as to reap the wonderful rewards of doing better. The greatest reward, even above bringing about great changes in our health, is being able to help others. Daily, we get to help people know better so they can do better. It is a win-win situation for everyone.

You are receiving this information for a reason. Are you content with your health? Have you just received a diagnosis that you're unwilling to live with? Are you tired of the burden of overweight or obesity? Are you tired of the struggle? Are you ready to be able to share a long, happy, healthy life with your family and friends? Are you ready to go to the next level?

If you have reached a tipping point and are looking for information, I encourage you to learn what we have to offer. In the United States today, our overweight/obesity rate is at a record high of 70 percent — and, incredibly, it continues to increase! This is not just an individual problem; it's a problem for the well-being of our entire nation.

Weight loss is a huge business in the US. My question still remains: If the solutions we are offered were working, why is obesity still a huge problem? Why do the people I now coach report having struggled all their lives, some for over sixty years? When we spend countless billions looking for solutions, shouldn't we have eradicated this problem?

I had a lifelong struggle with excessive weight. My appendix and gall bladder were removed — problems that were directly rooted in my obesity. In junior high, I went to Weight Watchers, but that wasn't my solution. After I married, I lost forty-five pounds on Weight Watchers, and to keep it off I lectured and conducted meetings for two and a half years. It seemed that I was always "watching" my weight go up and down. I also led Weigh Down Workshop meetings and had many gym memberships over the years. With everything I did, I got just enough results to keep me going, but it was always a roller-coaster ride.

I didn't see that life of struggle as a limitation. I continued to do what I wanted. I wasn't sick or on any medications. I was able to be there for my family, and enjoyed that very much. I had closets full of clothes, grouped by "skinny," "not so fat," "fat," and "fattest" instead of clothes of consistent sizes grouped by seasons. When you're in the struggle you just do what you do. I lived most of my life on a low-fat 1,200-calorie regimen of artificial diet foods. A home economist, I was teaching the next generation how to eat healthily. In good conscience, I taught them about highly processed convenience foods. I passed along what I had been taught and what was in the books. It had nothing to do with health. I was a young, newly married woman who desperately wanted to experience pregnancy and raising babies. I wasn't healthy enough to get pregnant, and the times I did ended in early miscarriage. I didn't know better, so I couldn't do better. Don't get me wrong: I was a happy person. I was raising my three wonderful adopted children and I enjoyed life.

The things I did kept me from weighing 300-plus pounds and having high blood pressure or diabetes. I'm thankful for Weight Watchers and gym memberships. I was content at that level. I was back on the bench watching others play the game. I was happy to travel to family activities and watch my husband and kids play. After all, because of my weight, I spent most of my life on the bench cheering for others.

In the process of looking for solutions to help patients better their health, my solutions were revealed. Seven years ago, when we opened our chiropractic clinic, we thought we had the answer for everyone. During the first year of practice, we watched many people become free from pain and other health limitations, but there was a group of people who didn't get the dramatic, positive results that we knew were available. Why did some get amazing results while others just got satisfactory ones? When we grouped these people to see if we could find a common link, we noticed that those with limited results were overweight, middle-aged women. Overfed and undernourished, they were going, going, going, doing for everyone else, and sacrificing themselves. Like me, they enjoyed being on the bench cheering for their families and friends while gradually sacrificing their own health.

It's common to be content where we are, stuck in behavior patterns. We're so busy doing what we do that we don't take the time to look for better options. I was content in my obesity, comfortable in the struggle. After all, there were people who were much worse off. I was only seventy-five pounds overweight. I had no diseases, and I just took over-the-counter medications when I had a problem, which in retrospect was quite often. I used up all my sick days every year, but isn't that why we have them? Everything looked great from the bench of life.

I am so thankful to Walter Scott, our representative from Standard Process, the brand of whole-food supplements we use and recommend to patients. While at a conference, Walter gave my husband a copy of a book by Lorrie Medford, C.N. *Why Do I Feel So Lousy?* proved to be a tremendous blessing. After reading that wonderful little book, I knew better and could do better. We started working on the principles Medford taught. We followed the Standard Process purification process she recommended. I was off the bench and becoming the star player in my own life!

This was a springboard; for the first time in years, I felt good and was actively learning about the next level. We reaped many blessings that just a short time prior we hadn't even known existed. The cycle was broken and the search for more information was on! We bought countless books about whole foods, natural health, water, detoxification, raw foods, and many other subjects. We attended every seminar we could find that could help us navigate in this new world. We went repeatedly to many of the meetings Standard Process sponsored. Our level of health changed drastically over the first year. I went from a tight size 18 to a comfortable size 12. I was wearing misses' sizes and no longer had to buy women's sizes. Our cholesterol and triglyceride levels were in healthy ranges. We finally had an answer to our struggle. Many people benefited from our new level of awareness and our experiments on ourselves. My mom and dad improved their health as well. We loved living at this higher level and playing this game.

In the discovery process, we became familiar with the many problems created by the Standard American Diet (SAD) — the very same information I'd spent years learning and teaching to future generations. We learned the dire consequences of the processed foods we'd been eating. It was also evident why we were so overfed yet still undernourished. I developed a special interest in the hazards of the chemicals and preservatives added to our common convenience foods. In these years of study, I became aware of the chemicals in our cleaning products, body-care products, and make-up. These endocrine disruptors were wreaking havoc in my body. The awful menstrual cycles and infertility now had an identifiable cause. I could see clearly how consuming 1,200-calories of low-fat, artificial, highly processed foods had contributed to my many health difficulties.

I saw a much bigger picture. The more I knew the more I wanted to know. I was angry, I was sad, and there was no going back. Had I known these things sooner, what might have been different? What blessings did we miss? Could I have experienced a healthy pregnancy and have been able to raise a child who had my genes? How did this happen? Why did this happen? And above all, why wasn't something being done about these problems? I realized that I was the answer, at least for me and my family and anyone else who would listen. There was no choice. I couldn't continue practicing the fundamentals of the game of life. I had to get off the bench and get to work. I had to play the game. My life and the lives of those I cared about were at stake!

My story is far from over. I'm back in the game and playing full throttle! There's no reason why anyone should be content to sit on the bench of life. Each day I continue to learn, grow and improve my skills. I don't know how many levels there are to achieve. I know I'm going to keep going each day toward a higher level. The passionate little girl is back. Everything is fresh and new and full of possibility. I learned many lessons, and one day I hope we will be able to share them together. As you get ready to make your own life-altering moves, I hope you'll derive a morsel of hope from reading this book. Here are some things I'd like you to ponder as you evaluate where you are in the game of life.

Are you actually *in* the game? Are you content where you are, even if it's on the bench? There are many benefits of being in the game: You have people cheering for you, and a team to assist you. Once you've learned the skills at a higher level you can't easily go back. Have you ever tried to unlearn the alphabet? The basics are there, but where do you want to go? Use your team to pick you up. In the action of the game, I've seen many players who've fallen be helped up by another player. If you fell from the bench, who would bother to pick you up?

We must realize that this game of life is not all easy. Practice is needed. We will stumble. There will be growing pains and hurdles. People will disappoint us. But I promise you it is worth it!

Even though I spent much of my life on the bench, playing when convenient, the time has come for me to share. I don't wish for anyone the struggle I allowed in my life. There's a better way. I won't willingly sit out another minute of the game. I have a big job to do, and I'm ready and equipped for the challenge. There's no need for anyone to be bound to "normal" when we see a better way. The light my family always saw in me now shines brightly for others to see, no longer hidden in that uncomfortable, unproductive body. People are able to see my heart, and I am ready to help others shed pounds and inches and reveal their hearts as well.

You have probably already realized that I'm a passionate cheerleader. I'm here to tell you that you can be in the game and cheer for others at the same time. If your friends are not in your league, don't wait for them. Your job is to show the way and encourage them to work harder toward a higher level. Don't let anyone hold you back. You have greatness in you and others are depending on you to lead the way. We are all winners. We all came to win.

Chapter 9

My Knight in Shining Armor

Finding freedom is not a solitary process. It requires the help of others. In junior high when we were issued our locks, we weren't alone. We had a whole team trying to do the same thing. Finding our combinations was a group effort. Very often you would see two of us get together with our little slips of paper listing the combinations. When you try to do things alone it can just slow the process.

This is where I was blessed. I have my own knight in shining armor. For the last twenty-plus years my husband, Ben, has been by my side. He has ridden the roller coaster along with me. This was without a doubt part of my success in finding my combination to a healthy weight.

TLC Lean uses the concept of team support as a basic component. We know by our statistics that our Leaners are more successful when they attend the meetings for education and support. It has never failed: if someone was struggling with the program, he or she was not coming to class. The Leaners who never missed a meeting were the most successful.

Weekly support played a big part. Beyond that, we even saw some of our Leaners soar! What made the difference? They had a partner on the program. They had built-in daily accountability and support. This was common among our married couples. They worked on their combinations consistently. There was continual support and reinforcement of the new principles they learned.

We also saw the benefit of other partnerships. We had buddies who worked together, thus supporting each other in the workplace. Grandparents teamed with grandchildren. Whole families worked together. In our first group we had three generations in the program at the same time. That was a win-win all the way around. Talk about accountability! The exciting thing about that arrangement was that there were three great-grandchildren benefiting from the process. What a way to create new habits and lifestyles that impact future generations!

I was blessed to have built-in support while on my mission to find my very own combination. As you know, I had been on the roller coaster for a very long time. When Ben and I married, he wasn't overweight. He was working very hard in a job that required a lot of physical labor. He could eat just about anything and not gain weight. As our lives changed, so did that component. When he started his studies to become a chiropractor, the physical labor stopped, but his eating style remained the same.

During his many years of school, Ben's weight grew steadily along with mine. The lack of physical exercise was a big part of our increasing weight. The food we chose was also a major factor. Remember, Ben was carrying thirty or more hours a semester, and I was working three jobs to make ends meet. Our income was very limited. We struggled to get by, and the foods we bought were chosen for price and convenience — nutrition and health were not a priority.

Were we under some stress? The answer is a resounding YES! Does stress affect our weight and health? That would be another strong YES! We were fat and unhealthy to say the least. We had goals in mind, and we pushed forward, compromising our health along the way.

I remember going to Weight Watchers. I was a lifetime member. The first time I stepped on the scale and it read 184 pounds, I was devastated. A few years earlier, before starting Weight Watchers, I weighed only 178 at my heaviest. I thought that was horrible then. Now I, a former leader who'd always kept her weight around 140, had seemingly gained forty pounds overnight! How could this happen?

The sad thing is it didn't stop there. Over the next four years I bloomed to over 210 pounds. The highest weight on the scales was officially 212 pounds. The weighing stopped, because I couldn't bear the truth. By the fit of my size 18s, which were always stretched to the max, I could count on being over 220 pounds. Ben was right there with me at the same weight. We were definitely a team — we had supported each other into obesity! My knight could no longer fit into his shining armor.

While this shows the physical toll, it also illustrates the emotional, mental, and spiritual tolls. Stress was a huge factor. Our self-images had taken a beating. We were sick pretty often. Ben struggled with his studies. Caffeine and sugar were our drugs of choice. We were paying a high price. Our goal was to get him through school at all costs. He was going to be a chiropractor!

This is a situation common in the US today. We are the world's most overfed and undernourished country. We have the freedom to choose. We can achieve anything we set our minds on, but this drive is undermined by unhealthy habits. When healthy habits become lifestyles, we can cope much better, but Ben and I weren't there. Unfortunately, most of us aren't there.

We made it through. We had a chance to learn, and boy did we learn! Every time there was a chance to learn something that might help us find a piece of our combination, we were there. For seven years we've been on a mission together. We've read many books, listened to countless audio presentations, and traveled most weekends. It was worth it. Not everything we learned was beneficial, and we soon learned that it wasn't just one thing, but a lifestyle, a combination of habits and helps. Together we learned the basics and together we applied them. We soon were seeing progress. Alone we were sure to fail. It was crucial for us to find our plan and stick with it. We were strong because we were in it together.

We learned quickly that while some basic things applied to both of us, there were also some things that one might do successfully that weren't beneficial to the other. It seemed we were doing a dance of progress — two steps forward and one step back. We always saw enough progress to keep moving forward, though. The better we did, the more hope we had, and the more committed we became to learning and changing.

The two of us have shed a combined 135 pounds. Our trials were worth it. We also realize how important our mutual support was and still is every day. I am so thankful for the life we have. Although it was a struggle, I'm also thankful for the experience we shared at our unhealthy weights.

My knight in shining armor is now armed with health. Life is better all around. Living a healthy life at a healthy weight helps reduce the challenges. Stress is easier to deal with, and we're now equipped to help others on their journeys.

We're a good pair, and we've surrounded ourselves with an excellent support team. It's important on any journey to have a goal, and it's vital to have others to support that goal. Tell people about your goal, and ask them to join you on your journey. Surrounding yourself with a support team will increase your success and make it much more pleasurable.

The teamwork didn't end with Ben and me. We helped my parents learn some alternative choices, and they've changed their lifestyles as well. As our children and grandchildren see us model new behaviors and habits, they too benefit from these changes. Our siblings are welcoming changes too. Everyone benefits from a healthier lifestyle.

The benefit of the TLC Lean classes doesn't end when you complete the program. The Leaners build a whole community of support. Some become friends and check on each other. We may see each other at the grocery store, dining out, attending a ball game, or at some community event. It's very encouraging to see others living the "Leaning Lifestyle."

It's human nature to gravitate to others who support you and your interests. You could list your support group right now: they are a combination of friends and family. You have common interests and common lifestyles. Why not choose to create a healthy lifestyle for yourself and your family, and support that lifestyle by encouraging others and receiving their support in return?

Having my own knight in shining armor and my own loving supporters is amazing. Equally amazing is that the more love and support I provide, the more benefits reflect back to me.

Chapter 10

Trials Bring Triumph

We all have ups and downs. Some trials aren't even worth addressing, but some must be dealt with for us to move forward. Each person must face his or her own trials, and finding the combination to a healthy weight is no different.

There were two battles that were very important for me. Though they might not even be considerations for you, I'll discuss them to illustrate the inevitability of trials. Consider carefully which trials you can overlook, because they're often the ones that can sidetrack you from your goal. There's no point wasting precious time on your journey, so choose your battles wisely.

My two battles were complicated and took much time to understand and overcome. There are entire books dedicated to each of these trials. Learning and experimenting with the information provided by others is how I triumphed. I am thankful for these experiences; though not always easy or pleasant, they were beneficial to my well-being.

Having been a "good dieter" for so long, I celebrated many successes. I achieved a good weight many times over the years. The problem was that once I got off the diet, program, plan, or product of the moment, I'd quickly regain the weight.

One thing that plagued me when I was at a good weight was my midsection. Even when I was leading Weight Watchers and keeping my weight at goal, I still had no waist. I had small arms and legs, and my face looked drawn. My body composition was just not good. I would lose weight and get smaller, but my shape wouldn't change, so I still looked fat! I exercised, and the scales reflected the weight change, but it wasn't as visible at it should have been. My clothing sizes only changed a little because I remained so thick in the waist.

In 2004, Ben and I benefited from reading Lorrie Medford's *Why Do I Feel So Lousy?* The book accelerated our journey to find our healthy combinations. We were happy with our weight loss and we felt great. I was pleased to be down to 185 pounds, but continued to strive for better. Exercise was a daily routine. Up at 4:30 a.m., walking, lifting weights, and doing isometrics. The problem was that no matter what I did — eat healthily, work out consistently, and purify with foods and sauna — I was stuck at 185 pounds! For a year that was the story, so I stopped the early morning workouts that I really didn't enjoy. I continued to use the sauna and eat healthy foods. My weight still didn't change. So what had been the point of the morning routine? Apparently, there was none! I wasn't seeing any benefit.

In 2007, a possible answer to this frustrating dilemma became available. Kevin Trudeau's book, *Weight Loss Cures,* had just hit the market. I practically inhaled it one weekend while we were at a chiropractic meeting. What Trudeau wrote about made a lot of sense. I was already benefiting from most of the preparation he discussed — things like avoiding chemicals in foods, drinking certain teas, and eating specific foods.

The book also showcased the work of A.T.W. Simeons, M.D. Trudeau talked about how Simeons's protocol was very successful for weight loss. He referred to it as a cure. My interest was great. The book just highlighted the protocol. I would have to read Simeons's manuscript, *Pounds and Inches,* to get the full details. The problem was it used hCG, which he talked about as being hard to get. It required a prescription, and it was unavailable in the US at the time. My hopes crashed — so close, yet so far from victory. I wasn't going to take a shot of this "miracle something." I put away the book. After all, I was doing lots of healthy things.

Now let's fast-forward to 2009. I was happy living a life in a much healthier 185-pound body, and pleased to be comfortable in size-14 clothes. Sometimes I'd even find a size 12 that fit. Life was good. My weight had been stable for a long time, and pain or sickness was rare. My lifestyle was supporting my goals. I had decided that I was just designed to be a "bigger girl." Most people had no clue what I weighed. I concealed the extra with clothing, because it was all in my midsection.

My world and many other people's worlds were about to change. A patient whom we see only a few times a year came for a visit. He was a lot smaller, and had shed most of his weight in his midsection. We discussed what he had done. He was happy to share that he had followed Dr. Simeons's protocol. He also said that it was available without taking shots. I couldn't wait to find out more. I read Dr Simeons's manuscript. I knew this was an important factor in completing my combination. Freedom from obesity was once again a possibility.

I found a clinic in Oklahoma City where hCG in drops were

administered under the tongue. No shots! It was amazing how well it worked for me. The weight was melting away. I had a waist for the first time ever. My excitement was overwhelming. I thought I had found the "cure" just like Trudeau had written. My mind was on overdrive. This is a way I could help my family and others who'd struggled for so long.

Twenty pounds of abnormal body fat magically disappeared. I was wearing size 8 and sometimes even a 6 or 4. I had never been that small or shapely. I was excited, but also frustrated — frustrated with the process, not the result. When I went to the clinic to enroll in the ten-week program, they told me, "When you gain the weight back, you can do it again." What?! That wasn't what I had signed up for. I was looking for a cure, looking for freedom, not another roller-coaster ride!

The frustration wasn't that it didn't work, but that it did work just as Dr. Simeons had documented so many years ago. The frustration was that most people would never know the whole story. They would use hCG but not follow the procedures, have very limited success, and thus consider it a failure. Some who did the program would experience great results, similar to mine, yet be trapped on another unending ride. They would lose the weight, but because they hadn't changed their lifestyles, they would quickly regain it just like they would after any diet.

Dr. Simeons's work was remarkable. Hormone imbalances were no longer a problem for me. Because I'd already established a healthy lifestyle, freedom from obesity was finally mine. The combination was complete. I was released from the bondage of obesity. Time has proven this to be a fact. Freedom is still mine. I am living a healthy life at a healthy weight. Pain and sickness are not even a rare occurrence.

Frustration was still a burden, however. Few people were

going to do the reading and research needed to uncover the whole protocol, as I had. I wanted to help others experience this freedom. Too many people I loved were still trapped in overweight, unhealthy bodies. I continued to refine my lifestyle and health, and continued to search for a way to put together a program to help others.

My prayers were answered. In less than a month, I learned about Dr. Beth Golden who, like me, had spent many years struggling with weight issues. She had devoted a decade to her training, and had developed a complete and natural program. I was so thankful to find a program that would not only help people shed their excess weight but also help them develop lifestyle habits that would support a healthy weight.

We implemented the program for a year. One hundred twenty people joined the fourteen-week program. In one year, we documented the fact that over 2,500 lbs. of unwanted fat had disappeared. Before-and-after photos told the story. The results were consistent and expected. It was like a law: When people followed the protocol, they achieved amazing results; when they continued the lifestyle, they continued to reap rewards from their investment of time, effort, and resources.

Unfortunately, many people will not benefit from the work of Dr. Simeons, Dr. Golden, and others like them. So many people are still looking for that pill, potion, or product that will work magic. On the Internet, hCG is available at many different prices, and much confusion surrounds it. It saddens me to know how valuable hCG — done correctly and supported with lifestyle changes — could be for so many, yet so few will have this privilege.

When people ask me what I did to shed the weight, I hesitate to even mention hCG. So many people have tried it and have been unsuccessful or experienced only short-lived success. When asked what I did, I reply that it was a combination of things. I might mention my success with hCG, because it made a significant change. I often explain that hCG is like the final detailing on a car. Cleanup and repair are needed to gain the greatest benefits from hCG. The process is also of major importance. If you had a classic vehicle, you would carefully choose the proper wax and apply it with precision. Once the final detailing was done, you would treat your classic car with care.

I am very happy to observe that more and more people are taking responsibility for their health and are embracing change more easily. You are proving this by reading this book and others like it. More people now realize that the answers don't come from someone else and what they do to or for you. A greater number are turning away from the miracle pills, potions, and other products. Many have take charge of their own health by changing their habits and lifestyles. They are unlocking their own combinations to freedom.

The second trial I wish to share was brought to our attention by our grandson Kolby, who, though he is just five years old, has taught us a lifetime of lessons. Kolby is a very intelligent and loving boy. There's not much he can't do or won't try. He has always been independent and considerate of others. A few years ago our daughter started to become concerned with Kolby's behavior. Developmental delays were also starting to become very noticeable.

At times Kolby would become abnormally aggressive. He didn't react to pain. Sometimes he would be very destructive. We noticed that he was developing more slowly than others his age. This caused his parents considerable concern. Mostly they were concerned with his safety. He was tested for things such as ADD and autism, and was placed in a special program at school to help with speech and other delays.

Our daughter, Jenny, read and researched, seeking knowledge of what they could do to help Kolby. Wanting to avoid medicating him, they started eating more natural, whole foods. As Ben and I read and attended seminars while on our journey of healthy living, we too looked for tidbits to help Kolby.

A major breakthrough was the removal of gluten from his food choices. It has been amazing to watch him change. He has become much calmer, and is non-aggressive and not destructive when he doesn't eat gluten. He is making developmental milestones at a record pace. It still amazes us how his behavior can regress in an instant by eating just a small amount of gluten. Even at his young age, he wants to avoid gluten, because he doesn't like what happens when he eats it.

What has this to do with being free from obesity? Well, in support of Kolby we started consciously avoiding gluten. In our studies we saw how many people were affected, and in how many ways gluten sensitivity could affect them. I already knew that eating any food that contained gluten made the skin under my eyes become puffy.

During the process of shedding my weight, gluten-containing foods were not part of the plan. While I was reducing, I noticed no puffiness under my eyes, and coughing, mucus, and bloating were gone. I didn't eat wheat, barley, rye, spelt, or oats very often. When I did occasionally eat them, it was worth the price of a little puffiness or a little mucus. After a weekend seminar on gluten sensitivity, however, we changed our minds. The devastation gluten could cause in the bodies of those sensitive to it seemed incredible. For two months we removed all gluten from our choices. It was an eye-opening experiment. Ben and I felt and looked better. This was not only a way to support Kolby but also a way to enhance our health.

Gluten-free living is a part of my freedom combination. We enjoyed the benefits by default while on the cleansing and reduction parts of our program. Now it's just a part of our lean lifestyle. It saddens us that Kolby ever had to struggle, but we're happy to know about the effects of gluten on our bodies.

Now that gluten is not among my food choices, my weight doesn't fluctuate very much. I don't get puffy or have to deal with gas or uncomfortable bloating. As more people discover that gluten is a problem for them, more gluten-free options have become available. Yes, you can eat cake and cookies, too! Try gluten-free eating for two months. Then have a day when you indulge in your favorite glutenous foods. If you are sensitive, what you feel will likely motivate you to say goodbye to gluten permanently.

If learning of these trials piques your interest, do your own research. You'll find it worthwhile. If you don't want to spend the time, learn from someone who's already triumphed. This advice applies to other trials you may encounter as well. Remember, trials will come, but you deserve to be victorious!

Chapter 11

My Secret Stronghold

Often, things are not as they appear. As you have read, being overweight is not just a physical weight problem. It can be quite complex in nature. Those who are burdened with excess weight understand the physical bondage. Most likely they understand the emotional trials as well. Mentally, the battle is constant, and the spiritual consequences are very costly. By now I hope you see what a multifaceted issue obesity really is, and understand why there's no a pill, potion, product, or program that will fix it all.

It's uplifting to realize that we do have control. We can control our thoughts and our words and emotions. We can control what we eat and what we allow in our environment. We can control whom and what we listen to. We can choose our activities, and choose what products and programs we buy and use to help us. The thing we most often forget is that we are in control. We hold our combination locks firmly in our own hands. We have the freedom to learn and to make educated decisions. We are free to make mistakes, and free to not give up after trying. We are even free to not try at all.

Just as back in junior high, each of us must accept the lock he or she was given. It's not much different from any of the other locks. They look alike, yet each combination is uniquely different — it is our own. Everything we need to successfully open and reopen our lock is available to us. We have resources that allow us to learn to do so with ease. At some point we don't even think about opening our locks; it becomes so routine that we can just let our fingers work the combination naturally, just like all our habits that we reinforce daily.

Everything we need to be free from obesity is within us or around us. If it doesn't seem so at first, just wait, it will become available. Timing is important. Had I learned about Dr. Simeons's work years ago, it would have been less beneficial because I wouldn't have had my lifestyle in place. I would have stayed on the never-ending roller coaster. Finding the proper sequence is also important. There's no point in waxing a dirty car. Although the solution may seem distant, I assure you it is available for you.

I hope you know by now how much I want you to have freedom from obesity — and from any health issue, for that matter. My goal is to give you hope. It's really not that difficult, though it can be complex. Remember: it's a journey. Think of it as a vacation, a permanent vacation in a beautiful place. Freedom is worth it. You are worth it. Though there will be trials, you can triumph, because you have a greater understanding and are surrounding yourself with a great support system.

The human body is incredible. It is fearfully and wonderfully made. No machine even comes close to its capabilities. All the computers and technology available to us today combined pale in comparison. Somewhere along the line we seem to have forgotten this. Like a computer, your body has memory. Science has shown that each cell of your body stores memory. When we are able to understand this we can tap into our power to change. We have touched on it only a little with our language, thoughts, and emotions.

Your body is designed to be a shelter, a vehicle, and a temple, and it is equipped to serve you all your life. It will protect you at all costs. When I started to understand this, my life changed. When I realized that my body was designed to protect my life, it rocked my world. Instead of being frustrated with how it looked and worked, I started to care for my body differently. When I had an ache or pain, I viewed it as a signal instead of covering it up with a painkiller. I would consider, "Why am I in pain?" I would ask, "What must I change for that alarm to be unneeded?" For so long I turned off or covered up the warning and continued to have the same problem.

Look at it this way: Would you ever hit your thumb with a hammer and then bandage it or take an aspirin and proceed to hit your thumb again? Is it helpful to cut the wires on your vehicle's CHECK ENGINE light so it's no longer a nuisance? Isn't that exactly what we do when we get a warning signal from our body? We should stop to ask, "Why do I have a fever?" or "Why this pain?"

When people come to our center, I often tell them to be thankful for the pain. Yes, that is very difficult, but consider this: were it not for pain, we might not have our fingers. We would surely have burned them off or cut them off by now. Pain is our STOP sign. We should heed.

Parents understand this. They don't want to cause their children pain, but sometimes a young child needs to feel a little pain. Parents can see their children are headed for trouble and spank them to redirect them. We even see this process in nature. A mama dog will nip at her pups' heels to get them out of harm's way. In truth, receiving painful correction has saved many of our lives.

I am going to share what I consider my "secret stronghold." I'm not sharing it because I want you to share in my sorrow, but so that you can see the depth of the bondage some of us experience. There are many who have much heavier burdens to carry; this just happens to be mine. My hope is you can face your secret stronghold and release your burden. Our burdens can be very heavy, and we often support them with habits and lifestyles that manifest as obesity and other health issues.

I love my body now that I'm free from obesity. Is it perfect? No. Can I continue to change? Yes. The area I continue to work on pertains to my "secret stronghold," which is a very emotionally charged issue for me. Because these issues can entail such powerful emotions, I encourage you to find someone who can help you uncover and let go of these emotions. Remember, your help comes both from within you and around you. It's wise to let others help. You have a support team for a reason. Don't struggle alone.

At the time of this writing I still have twenty pounds that could be released from my body. That weight is concentrated in my belly. The hCG helped me let go of most of my midsection, and the removal of gluten has eliminated abdominal bloating. Even with all that, I still have a round belly.

If I wear certain types of clothing, my belly is very noticeable. Over the years, many people who didn't know have asked if I was pregnant. For this reason I'm very careful what clothes I choose to wear. Why does that matter? How could that be a stronghold? If you recall, I do have three children who became mine through adoption. I am very thankful to have been allowed to be their mother. I want everyone to know how blessed I am to have them in my life.

Despite all the love I share with my children and grandchildren, there is something missing. There is a great desire I hold on to, a lack that I deal with daily. As long as I can remember, all I wanted was to be a mother. I wanted to experience the nine months of pregnancy. I yearned to carry a life in my body. I hoped to deliver into this world someone with my genes. I looked forward to the bonding of family that surrounded a new birth. My talents are in nurturing and teaching — vital skills for mothers. As soon as Ben and I married, I did everything I could to prepare for a healthy pregnancy. When it didn't occur, I found an infertility specialist to help.

This was the most emotional period of my life. Between my already deep desire and the hormonal fluctuations caused by fertility drugs, I was an emotional mess. I conceived twice. Both were tubal pregnancies that ended in early miscarriage and required emergency medical care. Like my struggle with obesity, this too was an extremely emotional ride. It was more like a fierce tornado, spinning at high velocity.

Today, this storm still rages. My desire for pregnancy persists. Monthly, it comes in hope and ends in disappointment. Though short-lived and not as strong, the desire is ever present, and my small round belly is a constant reminder. This is my stronghold. Someday I will be free from its grip. I see progress as time passes. Just acknowledging it as my stronghold has helped. Someday soon, I hope to announce I have delivered my stronghold. When this time comes, I expect the little round belly will be gone. I expect the scales to report a release of those final twenty pounds that I've held so closely for so long.

When this time comes, I'll be totally and completely free from obesity. At this point I'm free, but still carry some little reminders of the past bondage. I guess it could be considered *bondage baggage.* I must be ready to let those reminders go. I predict this final farewell to my remaining baggage is coming soon. But let me assure you that I am blissfully happy with my freedom and the healthy body I've been blessed with. Baggage or no baggage, I am free!

Do you have a secret stronghold? Is something keeping you on that endless ride? Are you seeing some of your combination to a healthy weight? I hope you'll discover what keeps you bound to that extra weight.

At first I was unaware of my secret stronghold, but as I worked on my combination to a healthy weight, understanding dawned when I grew ready. Proper timing, sequencing, and synergy all play a role in this process. Had my secret stronghold been visible to me from the start, I might have missed out on some of the other steps that helped me unlock my freedom.

At times this process can become frustrating, which is why I encourage you to find a support team. It pays to surround yourself with others who have similar goals, and to share your new habits and lifestyle with others who embrace similar ones. Once you uncover any secret strongholds, share them with your like-minded supporters. It will not only speed your progress, but it will help them as well. Uncovering secret strongholds is a positive step toward letting them go, and once you release your secret strongholds, freedom is within your grasp.

Chapter 12

The Master Key

It's not always easy to unlock a combination lock. The learning process can take a great deal of time when you're just beginning to learn how to dial the combination. Even with the combination written down, you can still have difficulty getting the lock to open. There is always a solution, however, a master key that will open all the locks. It was always good to know that there was one master key that would unlock every one of the locks for our gym lockers. That took some pressure off our minds while we were in the process of learning how to open our locks.

There is also a master key to freedom from obesity. This key will work on all locks, whether the bondage is obesity or any other health issue. The power of this master key is incredible. Once I discovered it and actively put it to daily use, it not only unlocked my freedom from the bondage of obesity, but also unlocked my freedom to an abundantly healthy life.

Having the master key firmly in my grasp took much pressure

off my mind and eased the struggle. All the highs, lows, and twisting turns of the dieting roller coaster were gone. The master key not only opened the lock of obesity, it unlocked the door of possibility. After forty years in bondage I was free. My whole life changed. I was able to make freedom lists like the one I shared with you earlier. I discovered a bountiful life, and this is where I live every day. It's fantastic that we can escape the limited life of obesity and other health issues, and live a healthy life full of possibility.

It brings me great pleasure to share the concept of the master key with you. Once you start using it, your answers will come and you'll discover your combination to a healthy weight. The "master key" is LOVE. Sound simple? It is. I always knew love was important. Love has surrounded me all my life. I showed love to others and received love daily. What I didn't know was how extremely powerful love really is. I had never before used love as the incredible tool it is. The longer I used this master key — the more I put the power of love and loving into focused practice — the greater my life became. As yet, I haven't found a lock it cannot open.

The master key has another amazing characteristic: The more it's copied the stronger it grows. This was very evident in our TLC Lean classes. We've already discussed the power of having a partner or a support team. Students were already using the master key. That's why it was easier for them to envision freedom and have a smoother journey. That's what made it easier for them to hold on to freedom and live healthier lives. They were using the master key, but had not yet discovered its awesome power. As much as I use my master key of love, I don't think I've tapped its full capacity.

In retrospect, being surrounded with love my entire life

kept me going. Remember: I was happy in my bondage. I had parents and other family and friends who loved me uncondi-tionally while I was in bondage. They even supported me in my captivity, because many were there with me. I enjoyed life, and didn't feel limited. I loved others and they loved me. I felt supported, comforted, and content. What I was missing was love of self. I liked myself but did not love myself. I never wanted to be selfish or self-centered. I didn't understand the difference between love of self and self-love. There's a big dif-ference. When you truly love something or someone you take care of it. You nurture it and care for it.

I see very clearly how my parents' and grandparents' love shaped my life. I am so very thankful for that unconditional love. When I began to love and care for me, things began to change for the better. When I started to give my body loving care because it was precious, my health began to improve. Think about how love has shaped your life. Think about the people who you've loved and those who have loved you. The power of love is around us all the time. It's always available, but for some reason we haven't tapped into it.

Ben, my knight in shining armor, helped me discover the power of unconditional love. For over twenty-one years the power of his love has influenced my life. Each day is better than the one before because of the love we share for each other. In me, Ben saw a person I didn't know. He saw beauty that I didn't see. He was able to uncover the person I had for so long concealed. The master key he used was love. It came packaged with understanding, encouragement, enthusiasm, and compassion. Every day, in many ways, he tells me I am his sweetheart. He loves me constantly and consistently. His love helped me see how precious I was. I knew how precious he and my family were to me, but I didn't see how loving myself could help me and my family. Love unlocked an amazing life for both of us.

Love is relentlessly creative. It helped us create unhealthy bodies while we were surviving school, because we were focused on school and survival instead of focusing on our bodies. Now it helps us daily to create vibrant, healthy bodies, because we focus love routinely on our health. The love Ben and I share with each other has helped us transform in many ways. I have supported him with love through all the ups and downs of school and starting and running a successful business. Without our total commitment to love each other unconditionally, none of our accomplishments would have been possible. We are thankful to know the power of love. We use it daily to improve our lives and the lives of others. My great desire is that many people will benefit from the love I share through the thoughts expressed in this book.

Ben and I first learned about the master key of love when we got married. As part of our wedding gift, a good friend gave us a story, copied from *Women's Day*, titled "Johnny Lingo's Eight Cow Wife." Widely available on the Internet, I've referenced it here because it describes perfectly for you how the master key works. Johnny saw his wife in a different light than everyone else did. He treated her as the beauty he saw, and she came to reflect that beauty for all to see. A few words from the story sum it up.

There are things that happen on the inside and things that happen on the outside. However, the thing that matters most is how she views herself. In Kiniwata, Sarita believed she was worth nothing. As a result, that's the value she projected. Now, she knows she is worth more than any other woman in the islands. It shows, doesn't it?

Love is a wondrous refining tool. We all use it daily, but not to its full capacity. We use its power but so we often misdirect it. We see love as limited. Please reinvestigate your thoughts about love. I hope you will rediscover the tremendous power you can use. It will be to all our benefit when we all claim the benefits of this unlimited gift. When you embrace this master key of love your life will transform before your very eyes. The things you want to change will change. The things that are harmful will disappear. The relationships and circumstances that contribute to your greatest good will increase.

A few years ago I chose to embrace this most bountiful gift of love. I decided to learn to properly care for the amazing body that was so lovingly designed for me. I devoted a full year to loving and caring for myself. It was a transformational year, during which I learned most of what I share with our students and in this book. To really make that year effective, I had to love Karen. I had to practice unconditional love toward myself. I was already committed to loving others unconditionally. Once I started to look at myself with love and focus on the positive, the transformation began. I started to see myself in a different light. I quickly realized that when I loved myself I could love others more. The boundaries that I had lived within for so long disappeared. Love is truly the master key.

Scripture talks about the gifts of faith, hope, and love. It refers to love as our greatest gift, and I wholeheartedly agree. Without love, hope and faith tend to disappear. Without love we are limited. When we don't love ourselves enough to take care of our precious bodies, we are in bondage to our own beliefs and the beliefs of those who surround us. My saving grace was to have been surrounded by many who loved me, who could look past my unloved body and see the person hidden inside. I am barely able to express my thankfulness for their love.

Now you see why I'm on a mission to help others who are ready to find their combination to a healthy weight. I urge you to first apply the master key and discover the benefits of loving and caring for your own body. Because love grows and expands rapidly, you'll be surprised at how fast your life can change as you find your freedom to a healthy weight. Once we start to duplicate this master key, the possibilities are endless. You will see the bondage of obesity disappear, and along with this freedom will come renewed health. My dream of living in a world where only 30 percent of our population is limited by their weight is alive and well.

You might think, *all this sounds good and I feel encouraged,* yet you're hesitant to get too excited. That master key may be visible but still past your grasp. Let's look at the experience you already have with love. We all love. There are people whom you love unconditionally. The ones it's easiest to love are our parents, spouses, and children. We also love our friends. Sadly, many of us love relationships, circumstances, and things more than we love ourselves. Once you grasp this master key you'll see that it's the ultimate win-win. When you love yourself you have more love to share with those you already love. Because of the expansion of this love you will also have more to share with others as you enjoy your more healthy body.

How do you grasp the master key? First, everyone is different, and everyone shares his or her love differently. The best way to evaluate whether you need to reprioritize a little and increase your love allowance for yourself is to sit down and look at how you spend your time, effort, and resources. We tend to allocate the most to what we love most. Think about your family. Don't you devote the majority of your time and energy to them? Are you and your health so far down on your priority list that you're only getting the crumbs? Isn't it time to break free from this bondage?

Such an evaluation is a self-exam. Only you know how you feel. You are the one who must look in the mirror. It's up to you to decide that you're worth the time, effort, and resources. When you can see past the barriers you've built over the years, reprioritizing will get easier and easier. A shift will happen. You'll see freedom on the horizon. You'll grasp the master key, and you'll soon enjoy health and have an abundance of love to share with others.

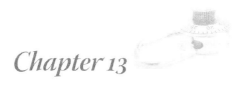

Chapter 13

The Power of One Hand

It is of great benefit to hold the master key, but it's also vital to know your own personal combination. Knowing how to release the lock confidently and consistently is the ultimate goal. Finding your combination to a healthy weight will take time and persistence to become reality. When you give yourself that time, life at a healthy weight will be yours.

I want to give you five principles that are basic to all our weight combinations. A good way to remember them is to envision holding these powerful principles in one hand. It's like unlocking your gym locker with one hand time and time again. My dad taught me the power of one hand. When I was three, he lost one hand in a farming accident. This has never been a limitation for him; there isn't anything he can't do with just one hand. So let's use the power of one hand to remind us of these five unlocking principles.

Look at your hand. Consider all of your fingers. Let's assign a principle to each. Once you know the principle assigned to each finger, I'll briefly explain how to apply them.

- ◆ Thumb — Show Up
- ◆ Index Finger — Clean Up
- ◆ Middle Finger — Straighten Up
- ◆ Ring Finger — Fuel Up
- ◆ Pinky — Link Up

Show Up — Extremely important to remember and apply, it has some common links with the master key. We tend to neglect ourselves, and it is reflected in how we care for ourselves. First you must show up and be present in your body. Showing up must be a daily activity. If you don't stay in charge of your body it will take the path of least resistance, which means it will likely deteriorate. Just like anything else, if you don't take care of your body intentionally, it will fall apart. Think about what happens to a house that isn't lived in. It starts to decline rapidly. I heard someone say once, "Our body is like a pet: the more attention it gets the better it will behave." Show up and pay attention to the health of your body. It is easy to focus on everything around you and neglect what's truly important. Make your health a priority by showing up each and every day.

A big part of showing up is looking at your body and assessing the situation. I know this can be painful, especially at first. To really show up you need to bare all. You must look at your body. You must listen to the words you are choosing, consider your thoughts, and acknowledge your emotions. If you don't know where you are, you limit your success. You must determine a starting point before any change can occur. You need to evaluate your status so you can make a plan.

Look at yourself privately. Take the time to make this analysis with no distractions. The best way is to look at your naked body in the mirror and ask yourself whether you're happy with the condition of your body. Over time, as you see progress, this will become easier; eventually you'll enjoy the gratifying transformation that's occurring. I also encourage you to weigh and measure. Keep a record of these numbers so you can track your success. Another great way is to take photos; these will serve as an encouraging tool as you make your journey.

Pay very close attention to your thoughts, feelings, and words. At first you may have to monitor them very closely. The body you're observing was created by your thoughts, feelings, and words. Keep these very positive so your actions and habits reveal the positive change you are showing up for. Be very cautious. Use this information objectively. It is important not to get stuck on the numbers or what you see reflected in your mirror. If you're feeling uncomfortable, be sure to take advantage of the master key of love. Your starting point is just a baseline. It all gets better from here when you show up.

Clean Up — This much-overlooked principle is applicable in many areas of life, yet we often neglect it when we consider the health of our bodies. We see the need to keep our homes clean, and we clean our vehicles inside and out. It's crucial to learn why cleanup is needed and how to incorporate it into your daily routine. In our TLC Lean classes, we spend at least a month learning clean-up techniques.

Our complete program includes tools that make the clean-up process easier, such as dry skin brushing, exfoliation, and far infrared sauna. Cleanup is vital for long-term health. It's highly beneficial during the reduction phase, and once you've done the initial cleanup and have established healthy habits, it will become an invaluable part of your healthy lifestyle. I look forward to using my clean-up tools and techniques every day.

Cleanup is not just a physical process but also a mental, spiritual, and emotional one. All negative thoughts, words, and feelings need to be deleted. Negativity delays success and causes struggle. Dump the need to be critical. Forgive yourself and others. It's time to detoxify from all doubt, fear, and excuses. Let go of the past so you can enjoy the abundance of health and well-being that's available.

Some things need to be cleaned daily, while some need to be cleaned only periodically. This is similar to changing the oil and filter in your car or doing a thorough spring cleaning in your home. At first these processes are new and will require a little extra effort, but over time they'll become a welcome habit. Our Leaners embrace the clean-up principle.

Straighten Up — One of my dad's favorite sayings is "A place for everything, and everything in its place." The older and more experienced I get the more I acknowledge the importance of this principle. When I was imprisoned in an obese body, everything seemed out of place. Here is another saying that applies: "Shape up or ship out." That's exactly what I did. Things were in such chaos that I just gave up and started focusing all my attention on those around me. I was out of alignment physically, emotionally, and spiritually.

The need to straighten up occupies our minds daily when it comes to our physical body. Being married to an upper cervical chiropractor and watching him address problems when bodily misalignment occurs gives me an enhanced perspective. We all know the importance of "having your head on straight." When the body is in proper physical alignment, everything works better. The brain can communicate more effectively with the rest of the body when our heads are on straight. When the body is out of balance and there is miscommunication at the brainstem, the body is limited. This can cause stress throughout the body, cause it to react to the stress, and thus limit its ability to express health.

Any time you can get your body to work together the greater the health benefits. Paying attention to posture is very beneficial. When you sit and stand up straight it takes unneeded stress off your body. Exercise is another super way to straighten up. Find things you enjoy doing so you incorporate exercise into your normal routine. The best exercise is the one you'll actually do!

It's also important to straighten up our thinking and our attitude. Many of us will find that we would benefit from an attitude adjustment. It is important to keep a positive attitude. *Stinking thinking* can limit our success. It's important to always have a success goal and to have reward markers to focus on as you make this journey. When you're looking toward your health goals it's easier to stay on course. From time to time you'll have to correct course and straighten up, but it won't be so difficult when you're focused on the goal ahead.

One of the great benefits of our TLC Lean classes is that healthy weight goals are clearly defined and a plan is in place. Everyone knows his or her plan, and they all have support and encouragement when they need to straighten up. Having a great support team in place helps us straighten up instead of giving up.

Fuel Up — How we choose to feed or fuel our bodies is extremely important. There is much confusion on how to do this. The dieting industry, with its low-calorie, nutrient-depleted foods, continues to contribute to our confusion, keeping us overfed yet undernourished. It's time we fueled up properly, and looked at our food as fuel instead of filler. When you think of your body as a vehicle it helps you see your food as fuel. There are many different types of fuel. You wouldn't put gasoline in a rocket ship, nor would you put jet fuel into a car. The TLC Lean program helps Leaners learn the essentials of fueling their bodies properly.

One way to get back to basics is to choose foods based on their closeness to how they are in nature. Ideally, we would eat foods that we grew ourselves. We'd pick fruit from the plant or pick the plant and eat it raw. This is not realistic for most of us today, so we must lean toward as natural a diet as possible. Eat foods that God designed as food for your body. Focus on feeding your body nourishing fresh fruits, vegetables, nuts, seeds, and lean meats that have been raised without damaging hormones or other chemicals. We don't live in a perfect world, so it's important to make good choices. Over time, with more knowledge and understanding, you can make better choices.

It's important to keep it simple. Take baby steps. Try new fruits and vegetables. Include a great variety in your choices. Try new recipes and combinations. This will help you stay on track and keep you from giving up. Do all you can to fuel up the best you can. Avoid processed foods. Choose foods that don't come in cans, jars, bags, and other packaging. The more they are altered and processed, the less valuable they are as fuel for your wonderful body. When you fuel up with good nutrition, you feel better and look better. Getting plenty of good fuel and water provides us with abundant energy. When we are properly nourished our bodies become naturally lean and healthy.

Link up — I can't overemphasize the need to link up with others for success. By now you understand the importance of a support team. To be successful for the rest of your life and live at a healthy weight it's crucial to link up with those who will support your goals. Find others who are seeking freedom at a healthy weight. Finding the right people to link up with might be a challenge, but it will be worth it.

If you look at your family and friends, you will likely see that you tend to have similar interests, habits, and health status. If you are linked up only with others who are struggling with weight and health issues, you will most likely continue to struggle. Look around and find others seeking freedom at a healthy weight and link up with them. Find people who are living at a healthy weight and link up. Find a mentor or coach and link up. Success breeds success, so set yourself up to succeed. If you intend to live a life free from obesity, you must see it and feel it.

Learn to talk the talk and walk the walk. Look for people who aren't struggling with their weight and health. Observe and emulate what they do. Choose wisely whom you link up with — your success depends on it.

When you apply the master key of love and the power you hold in your hand, freedom is within your grasp.

Chapter 14

Forever Free

Forever is a long time. When we use this word, I wonder if we really understand it. We often say things like "I will love you forever" and "best friends forever." Do we really mean forever? Doesn't forever imply commitment? Many people fear commitment. We've all seen marriages whose vows included "together forever" but ended in divorce. The commitment that's implied when we say *forever* is often diluted or even omitted. When I state, "I'm free from obesity," I mean it from the bottom of my heart. I understand and embrace commitment. This also means I'm totally committed to freedom forever.

Committing to achieve freedom from obesity is worth the effort. The journey can be pleasurable. Each victory is thrilling. Each tiny step leads to another, and soon you can see freedom within your reach. Before long you've unlocked your combination to a healthy weight and have begun to experience true freedom. When you apply these basic principles, freedom is yours — and it can be forever.

When your *why* is big and visible, commitment comes easily. When I married Ben, commitment was no problem. I knew my why, and it remains visible and active today. The benefits of commitment are valuable. I like to say I come from a long line of love. My grandparents were married seventy-three years, and my parents will soon celebrate fifty years of marriage. Commitment comes easily when the master key of love is the *why*. Unconditional love is essential to make anything last forever.

When we are trapped on the unending diet roller coaster and experiencing all the problems it brings into our lives, we don't have a why. It takes no commitment to find ourselves captive in unhealthy bodies. When we don't have a commitment to ourselves and to our health, or have a big why, we end up on the path of least resistance. We forget how valuable and precious we are. This is a comfortable place because it's so familiar.

My purpose in writing this book is to offer hope, to communicate and demonstrate how living free at a healthy weight is possible and can last forever. Finding your combination to a healthy weight is a journey — often a total change of direction. A new vision is required along with a positive attitude. With a little love and some habit and lifestyle changes the phenomenal transformation can occur.

My journey as a free agent will never end. There will be ups and downs. When I have doubts, I look at my freedom list. This reminds me to stay the course. I always have a visual available of the body that represents health. I also keep a photo of the unhealthy body as a reminder of where I've been and never want to go again. Though painful to look at, it also reminds me of the rewards of staying on course with a healthy lifestyle.

I know how important it is to surround myself with a great support network. This includes other Leaners and those who know how important it is to me to live at a healthy weight. I guard myself from thoughts and language that might lead me back to the roller coaster. I am very proactive with my habits and lifestyle. When making food and activity choices, I evaluate whether they'll be beneficial and supportive of my healthy lifestyle.

This may require a lot of time and effort. It is worth it. Think about it. You are going to put your time and effort into something. Wouldn't it be better to spend that time on your well-being? In the long run, you will save time and effort because you made wise choices. When you're healthy you'll also save a lot of money. Being sick is extremely costly, and being limited by extra weight is painful. Freedom from obesity is entirely worth the investment of time, effort, and money.

It's crucial that you stay positive as you make this journey of a lifetime. You are the only one in control of your destiny. Others are available to encourage and support you, but the journey is yours. You may have a sweetheart or a knight in shining armor beside you all the way, but you are in charge of your choices. You must take each step. You determine the direction you take. You choose how much time, effort, and resources you'll dedicate to your freedom. In the end the reward for success or failure is all yours. Others will be affected, but you'll be affected by the result each and every moment.

It's also essential that you stay aware and committed to moving forward toward freedom from obesity and health difficulties. When you have stayed the path and gained your freedom, you want to hold on to it. This can be a struggle, so I want to alert you to a problem that troubles many: how to retain freedom forever. If you are aware of this, and of how devastating it can be, you'll be prepared to win the battle.

There is a state correctional facility housed in my hometown. All my life I've heard stories about inmates who had to return soon after gaining their freedom. Some would even sabotage their release by violating the rules just a few days before it was scheduled. I've watched the same thing happen to those who experience freedom from obesity. You might be thinking, *no way, not me.* Be careful! Remember: this is a forever journey — it never ends. Your experience can be either freedom or bondage — it can't be both.

I have the privilege of helping people from all walks of life. It is a great joy to learn from them. I found some interesting information that pertains to drug offenders, which I believe applies to our purpose. From their personal experience and expectations, counselors in the field have told me that a drug offender who has been confined for at least three years is most likely to be incarcerated again. Of those who receive treatment, only 20-25 percent are expected to live their lives in freedom. If no treatment is received, only 5 percent are expected to retain their freedom. What concerns the counselors most is the 3 percent who have cleaned up while confined and under care, yet return to drugs and die of overdose.

The same thing is happening with our health. When you've been on the diet roller coaster most of your life, it's so easy to return to what you know. One destructive choice leads to another, and it's then tempting to turn to the newest diet pill, program, or product. The statistics are grim. The overweight/obesity rates are similar to those of drug offenders. Only 20-25 percent of our population lives at a healthy weight. This should get our attention!

You might well wonder how this could happen, how someone could work so hard for freedom and then just throw it away. For some people, freedom can be scary. If you've spent most of your life in an overweight, unhealthy body, that situation is comfortably familiar. It's not optimal, but you know how to manage life under those conditions. Stepping into the unknown is scary. Remember: Many people have struggled with their weight for decades. They have learned the habits of struggle, and can live this life automatically. To keep their freedom they must be aware of their choices and live with intention. For many, it's a totally new and very frightening experience.

What's really scary, though, is the path that nearly 80 percent of our population is traveling: the bondage of obesity that is destroying both young and old. The journey is one of degeneration, ill health, disease, and premature death. You may be uncomfortable with my frankness, but love is not just gentle and kind; love is strong and bold. From the beginning I have shared with you from all the love in my heart. Now is no different.

Just as a mother dog nips at her pups to steer them away from harm, my intention is to guide you away from the danger and devastation. I want you to reap the benefits enjoyed by the healthy minority. The journey of the majority is guiding the whole at this point. It's time to change that direction.

This is a problem no one is immune to. Our individual health affects the health of the whole. When individual health is ruined, families are destroyed, and in turn entire communities are damaged. Obesity is also needlessly depleting our country's resources.

If we continue to do what we have always done, we will continue to get what we have always got. Plain and simple, isn't it? I was unhappy living in an unhealthy, obese body, so I made changes. I encourage you to make changes to improve your health. These positive choices will not only give you better health but also bring abundance to your life. Making the choice to seek freedom from obesity not only affects you but those around you.

My dream is to live in a world where no one must struggle with weight and health issues. This is possible. First we must take control of our own health, and then show others the way. The joy of living life at a healthy weight is contagious.

It is with great joy that I live at a healthy weight. I'm truly thankful for my life's journey — all of it, even the forty years of bondage. The contrast has deepened my appreciation. Every day I give thanks for another day to live in an amazing body that is resilient and can recover from poor decisions. Because of this appreciation, I am sharing hope of freedom each and every day.

This is why I've written of my journey. If I just help one mother see her worth and discover a better way to live and take care of her family; if I convey to one grandparent how important it is to share his or her hopes and dreams at a family table filled with fresh, healthy food; if I can show one child the importance of lovingly caring for his or her amazing body; if I can ignite just one spark of hope for a healthier future, my time has been well spent.

My journey is not complete, and neither is yours. I will continue to spread the news of forever freedom. I'll write more books, more lessons will be taught and learned, and health will continue to increase, all because I'm living free from obesity. I hope you'll join me on this journey. Together we can see all our dreams come true. What an amazing world it will be when we all live forever free!

About the Author

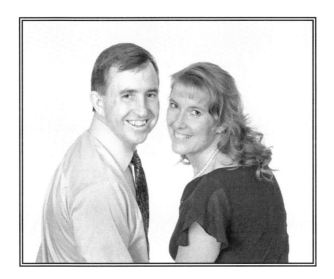

Karen Warren Locklear, founder of TLC Lean, is an inspiring advocate for thousands of people who desire to become "Free from Obesity". Karen is an enthusiastic team leader and has coached hundreds of people to reclaim their lean and beautiful figures. With her husband, Dr. Ben Locklear, she is also co-founder of TLC for Life — a state-of-the-art wellness center which specializes in leading people toward optimal health and wellbeing.